5

RECENT ADVANCES IN HEMATOLOGY RESEARCH

PLASMAPHERESIS AND INTRAVENOUS IMMUNOGLOBIN

CLINICAL USES, POTENTIAL COMPLICATIONS AND LONG-TERM HEALTH EFFECTS

Recent Advances in Hematology Research

Additional books in this series can be found on Nova's website under the Series tab.

Additional e-books in this series can be found on Nova's website under the e-book tab.

RECENT ADVANCES IN HEMATOLOGY RESEARCH

PLASMAPHERESIS AND INTRAVENOUS IMMUNOGLOBIN

CLINICAL USES, POTENTIAL COMPLICATIONS AND LONG-TERM HEALTH EFFECTS

ROSSANA ALLEGRO
EDITOR

New York

For permission to use material from this book please contact us:
Telephone 631-231-7269; Fax 631-231-8175
Web Site: http://www.novapublishers.com

Library of Congress Cataloging-in-Publication Data

ISBN: 978-1-63117-916-7

Library of Congress Control Number: 2014938431

Published by Nova Science Publishers, Inc. † New York

CONTENTS

PREFACE

Plasmapheresis is a therapeutic tool used to treat a wide range of disease processes, and in which the priority aim is to ensure sufficient plasma exchange to reduce or eliminate symptoms resulting from the action of pathogenic elements vehiculized in the plasma. Scientific selective apheresis with principles of evidence-based medicine involves the application of one of the oldest therapeutic modalities (bleeding), widely used between the fourth century B.C. and the second industrial revolution. This book provides information on the use of plasmaoheresis during pregnancy; therapeutic use of autologous plasma for the treatment of dry eye disease; and therapeutic plasma exchange in the neurological setting. It also discusses intravenous immunoglobulins. During the past decades intravenous immunoglobulins (IVIG) have gained more and more popularity for the treatment of a wide range of diseases and conditions. This treatment is extensively used in immune deficits, autoimmune thrombocytopenia, Kawasaki's disease, for the prevention of infectious complications due to hypogammaglobulinaemia secondary to myeloma, chronic lymphatic leukaemia and post-bone marrow and stem cell transplantation, in Guillain-Barre syndrome, etc. IV-Ig is obtained from the plasma of healthy blood donors and contains normal, polyclonal, polyspecific immunoglobins (Ig), mostly consisting of intact IgG. These antibodies are directed against non-self antigens, self-antigens (natural autoantibodies), and other antibodies (idiotypic antibodies). The administration of intravenous immunoglobulin (IVIG) is generally safe and well tolerated. However, the treatment of autoimmune disorders usually requires high dose therapy (1-2 g/kg) that may result in a greater frequency of side effects and adverse events. This book discusses several topics including the clinical application of intravenous immunoglobulins in autoimmune mediated ocular inflammatory diseases; complications of intravenous immunoglobulin therapy; clinical uses; and side effects.

Chapter 1 - The purpose of this chapter is to highlight the proposed mechanisms of Intravenous Immunoglobulin (IV-Ig) in the clinical application for treating ocular inflammatory disease. Corticosteroid sparing therapies for recalcitrant uveitis treatment are desperately needed, as corticosteroid monotherapy is wholly inappropriate for management of these patients, and no therapy is currently approved. Although not completely understood, IV-Ig acts through the mediation and/or regulation of multiple immune pathways, providing a widespread anti-inflammatory effect. Specific varieties of ocular inflammatory disease, namely ocular cicatricial pemphigoid, idiopathic uveitis, birdshot retinochoroiditis, retinal vasculitis, and scleritis, have the strongest collection of clinical data supporting the use of IV-Ig in patients failing to respond to therapy. IV-Ig is highly costly, resource-intensive, and carries a unique side effect profile. More research is needed to determine the future role of this therapy in the clinical setting.

Antibodies are an integral component of the immune system; found in blood, they act as surveillance proteins, protecting against infections, diseases, and malignancy in their host. In 1972, Gerald M. Edelman and Rodney R. Porter won the Nobel Prize in Physiology and Medicine for their discovery of the structure and function of antibodies, opening doors to new research in immunology and providing the information that led to immunoglobulin usage as clinical therapy (The Nobel Prize in Physiology or Medicine 1972, 2013).

Intravenous pooled immunoglobulin (IV-Ig) has found a place in the clinic as a therapeutic option in various diseases of the immune system. IV-Ig is obtained from the plasma of healthy blood donors and contains normal, polyclonal, polyspecific immunoglobins (Ig), mostly consisting of intact IgG. These antibodies are directed against non-self antigens, self-antigens (natural autoantibodies), and other antibodies (idiotypic antibodies) (A. Durandy, 2009). Originally, IV-Ig was employed as replacement therapy in patients with immunodeficiencies. In 1981, Imbach et al. were the first to report the favorable outcomes on children with immune thrombocytopenia by high dose IV-Ig therapy (Richter, 1995) (Imbach, 1981). Subsequently, IV-Ig treatment was trialed in a variety of other autoimmune disorders. In 1989, Sunakawa reported one of the first cases of beneficial effects of IV-Ig therapy in ocular inflammatory disease. The case described a patient with severe uveitis treated with high-dose corticosteroids, whose visual acuity (VA) was gradually deteriorating. After receiving two courses of IV-Ig, the patient's VA improved, and retinal exudation and phlebitis diminished (Sunakawa, 1989) (Tellier, 2005).

Several mechanisms have been hypothesized for IV-Ig's mode of action. IV-Ig interacts at multiple levels with the immune system, which include the following: (a) blockage and modulation of the expression of IgG Fc fragment receptors on the surface of macrophages; (b) modulation of the activated complement system; (c) modulation of cytokine synthesis and release; (d) modulation of cell proliferation, migration, and apoptosis; (e) modulation of B and T lymphocytes; (f) blockage and modulation of neutrophil cell activation and proliferation; (g) neutralization of circulating autoantibodies; (h) interaction with other B and T lymphocyte surface molecules (Tellier, 2007). The beneficial properties of IV-Ig last beyond the half-life of IgG, providing evidence that the effects are more than a mere passive neutralization of pathogenic autoantibodies (A. Durandy, 2009) (S.V. Kaveri, 2011).

A complete understanding of its role in immunomodulation is yet to be elucidated. Further research into the precise mechanisms of IV-Ig, with an emphasis on autoimmune diseases will eventually lead to a thorough understanding of IV-Ig.

The purpose of this chapter is to highlight the proposed mechanisms of IV-Ig, recognize their beneficial role in the treatment of ocular autoimmune diseases, and emphasize the importance of prioritizing investigations to study the possible, additional benefits IV-Ig has to offer.

Chapter 2 - The administration of intravenous immunoglobulin (IVIG) is generally safe and well tolerated. However, the treatment of autoimmune disorders usually requires high dose therapy (1-2 g/kg) that may result in a greater frequency of side effects and adverse events. These reactions may be generalized or specific to one organ. IVIG preparations differ in their excipients, physical characteristics (liquid versus powder), and chemical composition. The specific IVIG product administered therefore influences the type and severity of adverse reactions observed. The most common side effect is headache. Rarely, headache can be a symptom of aseptic meningitis. Some generalized reactions include fever, pruritus, rash, myalgia, arthralgia, and blood pressure alterations. These side effects can last for a few hours or several days. Thrombotic events, including acute myocardial infarction and stroke, have been reported with hyperosmolar products and may occur during or a few hours after administration. Acute kidney injury as a result of osmotic nephropathy is well recognized after infusion of sucrose containing IVIG products. The rise in creatinine occurs early after treatment and is reversible in most cases. The development of hemolytic anemia is a more recently recognized complication of high dose IVIG therapy. This is associated with non-lyophilized, liquid IVIG preparations which contain higher anti-blood group (A/B) antibody titers. There are also reports of acute kidney injury occurring as a consequence of pigment nephropathy as a consequence of hemolysis after IVIG administration. Lymphopenia and neutropenia may be detected after IVIG infusion. These cytopenias are self-limited and have not been associated with an increased risk of infection. Electrolyte abnormalities are also observed after IVIG therapy. The majority of cases manifest as pseudohyponatremia. However, true hyponatremia has also been reported. These disturbances usually go undetected and resolve without intervention, but can be clinically significant in the setting of renal insufficiency. Infusion reactions can be prevented by pre-medication with acetaminophen, diphenhydramine, and methylprednisolone. Acute kidney injury can be avoided by using non-sucrose containing products. However, these preparations contain higher anti-A/B titers and may result in an increased risk of hemolysis. Splitting the dose of IVIG and slower infusion rates can reduce adverse reactions. Using subcutaneous immune globulin may be effective for preventing some adverse reactions but this has not been effectively evaluated.

Chapter 3 - In this chapter the authors will review the diseases that most often require the use of plasma exchange therapy during pregnancy. It is well known the important role of plasmapheresis in the removal of the F-VIII multimers observed in the thrombotic thrombocytopenic purpura, but also the auto-antibodies that appear in autoimmune diseases like Myasthenia Gravis, Antiphospholipid Syndrome or Systemic Lupus Erythematosus. There are also some situations where plasma exchange therapy is being used recently with success like Isoinmunization, Gestational Penphigoid, Prymary Hypertriglyceridemia or Acute gravidic liver steatosis. Throughout this chapter the authors review the most important clinical and therapeutic features of these illness during pregnancy.

Chapter 4 - Dysregulation of T cell functions results in the development and maintenance of autoimmune and systemic inflammatory disorders. In this context, CD4+ (helper) and CD8+ (cytotoxic) T cell activation leads to autoantibody production and self-reactive cytotoxicity respectively. IVIg is commonly used as a second line immunosuppressive therapy in patients suffering from these disorders. Over the past decades, clinical observations in IVIg-treated patients revealed significant modulations in T cell populations and functions (Th1/Th2 ratio, Treg numbers, cytokine expression, etc.). Similar observations on the immunomodulatory effects of IVIg on T cell populations (e.g., activation and differentiation of various CD4+ subsets, reduction of CD8+ T cell cytotoxicity) were made using in vitro assays and animal models, suggesting that these experimental systems could be useful to decipher the mechanisms by which IVIg produces therapeutic effects in autoimmune and inflammatory disorders.

In this chapter, the authors will review the various effects of IVIg on T cells both in vitro and in vivo. The authors will also summarize the mechanisms proposed to explain these effects and discuss the reasons for the discrepancies between conclusions drawn from studies published during the last decades.

Chapter 5 - Eosinophilic granulomatosis with polyangiitis (EGPA; also known as Churg–Strauss Syndrome) is a rare disease characterized by allergic granulomatosis and necrotizing vasculitis following peripheral and tissue eosinophilia. The mortality and prognosis associated with EGPA are related to disease severity, as assessed by Five-Factor Scores; the survival rate at 5 years after myocardial involvement is reported to be one-third of that without myocardial involvement.

The mainstay of treatment for EGPA is systemic corticosteroid (CS) therapy. Additional treatments with immunosuppressive agents such as cyclophosphamide (CYC) or azathioprine may be helpful in some patients. However, mononeuritis multiplex or heart failure in some patients with EGPA or with antineutrophil cytoplasmic autoantibody (ANCA)-associated systemic vasculitis does not respond to combination therapy.

High-dose intravenous immunoglobulin (IVIG) therapy was effective against severe mononeuritis multiplex or heart failure in patients with EGPA that did not respond to combination therapy. IVIG treatment has thus shown clinical efficacy; it regulates the activation of T_{reg} cells in autoimmune and immune-mediated inflammatory diseases. Mechanisms implicated in IVIG modulation of T_{reg} function include activation and induction of T_{reg} cells by the Fc or $F(ab')_2$ domain of IVIG and enhancement of T_{reg} function by increasing the expression of FOXP3, TGF-β, IL-10, and CTLA-4. The authors confirmed that the number of T_{reg} cells is increased for at least two years after the last IVIG treatment. This finding could lead to a reduction in the maintenance dose of CS and suggests that IVIG therapy may improve the prognosis of EGPA patients with severe organ involvement.

However administration of IVIG alone, without concomitant treatment with CS and CYC as an initial treatment approach for EGPA, did not improve pulmonary infiltration or vasculitic symptoms in various organs, including the digestive tract and skin. Furthermore, it had no effect on peripheral nerve damage, cardiac dysfunction, or eosinophil numbers (including $CD69^{+}CCR3^{+}$-

activated eosinophils). Moreover, it is unclear whether the clinical and immunologic efficacy of IVIG is affected by the disease phase (e.g., during initial treatment or at relapse after remission). In addition, the characteristics of the patient's disease condition that influence whether remission is achieved after a single course or multiple courses of IVIG have not been assessed.

Chapter 6 - Intravenous immunoglobulin (IVIG) therapy has been used to treat several autoimmune or inflammatory diseases. The authors conducted a clinical trial of immunoglobulin therapy for acute myocarditis. The study consisted of the following: a comparison of prognosis between the patients treated with and those not treated with IVIG in multi-center study. 15 patients were treated with IVIG (1-2g/kg, over 2days), whereas 26 were untreated. There was a statistically significant difference between the survival curves of the patients treated with IVIG (20.0%, 3/15) and the survival curves of those not treated with IVIG (34.6%, 9/26). There was no significant difference between the IVIG-treated and untreated groups in terms of clinical parameters of acute and chronic phases. Therefore, therapy with IVIG seems to be a promising treatment for acute myocarditis given that it improves the clinical course.

Chapter 7 - Dry eye disease is a common ophthalmic condition that results from a complex interplay between tear production and the ocular surface, producing symptoms of discomfort, visual impairment, and tear film instability that can damage the ocular surface. Numerous treatment options for mild forms of dry eye disease exist, including lifestyle changes, artificial tears, tear secretagogues, and punctum plugging. More severe dry eye disease, however, is often unresponsive to conservative treatments because of the underlying damage to the ocular surface epi-thelium. The multitude of growth factors, cytokines, antimicrobials, and vitamins present in natural tears that normally supports the ocular surface epithelium is lacking in artificial tear solutions.

Blood-derived serum and plasma, however, contain many of the same components as the natural tear film and have been explored over the past decade as an alternative treatment option for patients who have failed more conventional treatments. Recent clinical trials have demonstrated the benefits of serum for dry eye disease and other ocular surface disorders, with improved patient symptoms, reduced ocular surface damage and improved healing. Trials using plasma prepared by plasma-pheresis have shown similar benefits, with the benefit of improved contamination control in plasmapheresis compared to standard serum preparation methods. In this chapter the authors discuss the current role of plasma in dry eye disease treatment, the use of plasmapheresis and related techniques for the preparation of treatment solutions, and the potential for future large-scale adoption of this method by clinicians and their patients.

Chapter 8 - During the past decades intravenous immunoglobulins (IVIG) have gained more and more popularity for the treatment of a wide range of diseases and conditions. This treatment is extensively used in immune deficits, autoimmune thrombocytopenia, Kawasaki's disease, for the prevention of infectious complications due to hypogammaglobulinaemia secondary to myeloma, chronic lymphatic leukaemia and post-bone marrow and stem cell transplantation, in Guillain-Barre syndrome, etc. Fewer studies have investigated the use of IVIG in patients with systemic lupus erythematosus (SLE), rheumatoid arthritis, dermatomyositis, multiple sclerosis, myasthenia gravis, in women with reproductive failure, etc.

The wide use of IVIG for the treatment of different diseases and conditions has lead to the emergence of multiple adverse reactions. The large majority of these side effects develop either immediately after the infusion, or within the next 24 hours: reactions at the site of administration (erythema and rash, itching), tachycardia and low blood pressure, nausea and vomiting, headache, joint and muscle pain, lower back pain, fever, hemolytic reactions, neutropenia, pulmonary edema, deep vein thromboses, etc. There are multiple causes for the development of these side effects, i.e., improper administration of IVIG for inappropriate patients/diseases, rapid intravenous infusion, large quantities of infused IVIG, lack of monitoring during the infusion, the presence of stabilizers and preservatives, sucrose, aggregates, small quantities of IgA or other biological substances and adulterants. An important factor for the prevention of these reactions is the strict attendance to the mode of administration of IVIG, the precise evaluation of the indications for IVIG treatment in every patient and the careful monitoring of the treatment in hospital conditions.

Chapter 9 - Therapeutic Plasma Exchange (TPE) is a therapeutic procedure in which blood of the patient is passed through a medical device, which separates plasma from the blood components. TPE is designed to remove or at least to reduce the concentration of (pathologic) large molecular weight substances from the plasma. The idea behind the procedure is that elimination of pathologic substances from the plasma reduces further physiological damage. TPE is mostly not a solitude therapeutic intervention to stop a pathological process, and is often accompanied with orally or intravenous drugs.

Therefore, it is interesting to know the pathologic substance, because it should be toxic, larger than 15000 Dalton, with a long half-life, to make removal by plasmapheresis instead of other eliminating techniques as hemofiltration or high-flux hemodialysis, valuable.

The best known indications in the neurological setting are Myastenia Gravis and Guillain Barré syndrome. When TPE is used in neurological disorders, there is not always certainty about the pathogenic substance that triggers the development of the disease. Mostly an autoimmune pathogenesis is suggested due to the presence of antibodies. The presumed antibody mediated tissue damage could probably interrupted by TPE.

Nowadays, evidence-based medicine is practiced and the ASFA guidelines promote therapeutic apheresis based on clinical data and controlled trials, rather than case reports. Indications are divided in different categories, based on evidence of clinical efficacy, ongoing from category I, disorders for which apheresis is accepted as first-line therapy, (for instance Guillain-Barré syndrome); category II for second-line therapy, (e.g., acute disseminated encephalomyelitis); category III, in which the role of apheresis is not confirmed (paraneoplastic neurologic syndrome) to category IV, including disorders for which apheresis should be ineffective or harmful. There is a separate category in which apheresis is only used in an experimental setting.

Although, the quality of evidence supporting the use of TPE in the treatment of most neurological diseases and disorders is often limited and many of the conditions are rare, it is unlikely that randomized controlled trials (RCT) will ever be performed. Therefore, the authors retrospectively examined all adult TPE-patients during a 7-year period (March 2005 - February 2012) and discovered some interesting observations.

In: Plasmapheresis and Intravenous … ISBN: 978-1-63117-916-7
Editor: Rossana Allegro

Chapter 1

Clinical Application of Intravenous Immunoglobulins in Autoimmune Mediated Ocular Inflammatory Diseases

Swetha Dhanireddy, MD[1,2], Jamie Lynne Metzinger, MS, MPH[1,2] and C. Stephen Foster, MD, FACS, FACR*[1,2,3]

[1]Massachusetts Eye Research and Surgery Institution, Cambridge, MA, US
[2]Ocular Immunology and Uveitis Foundation, Cambridge, MA, US
[3]Department of Ophthalmology, Harvard Medical School, Boston, MA, US

Abstract

The purpose of this chapter is to highlight the proposed mechanisms of Intravenous Immunoglobulin (IV-Ig) in the clinical application for treating ocular inflammatory disease. Corticosteroid sparing therapies for recalcitrant uveitis treatment are desperately needed, as corticosteroid monotherapy is wholly inappropriate for management of these patients, and no therapy is currently approved. Although not completely understood, IV-Ig acts through the mediation and/or regulation of

* Corresponding author: C. Stephen Foster, MD, FACS, FACR, Massachusetts Eye Research and Surgery Institution (MERSI), 5 Cambridge Center, 8th Floor, Cambridge, MA 02142 US, Tel: 617-621-6377, Fax: 617-494-1430, sfoster@mersi.com.

multiple immune pathways, providing a widespread anti-inflammatory effect. Specific varieties of ocular inflammatory disease, namely ocular cicatricial pemphigoid, idiopathic uveitis, birdshot retinochoroiditis, retinal vasculitis, and scleritis, have the strongest collection of clinical data supporting the use of IV-Ig in patients failing to respond to therapy. IV-Ig is highly costly, resource-intensive, and carries a unique side effect profile. More research is needed to determine the future role of this therapy in the clinical setting.

Antibodies are an integral component of the immune system; found in blood, they act as surveillance proteins, protecting against infections, diseases, and malignancy in their host. In 1972, Gerald M. Edelman and Rodney R. Porter won the Nobel Prize in Physiology and Medicine for their discovery of the structure and function of antibodies, opening doors to new research in immunology and providing the information that led to immunoglobulin usage as clinical therapy (The Nobel Prize in Physiology or Medicine 1972, 2013).

Intravenous pooled immunoglobulin (IV-Ig) has found a place in the clinic as a therapeutic option in various diseases of the immune system. IV-Ig is obtained from the plasma of healthy blood donors and contains normal, polyclonal, polyspecific immunoglobins (Ig), mostly consisting of intact IgG. These antibodies are directed against non-self antigens, self-antigens (natural autoantibodies), and other antibodies (idiotypic antibodies) (A. Durandy, 2009). Originally, IV-Ig was employed as replacement therapy in patients with immunodeficiencies. In 1981, Imbach et al. were the first to report the favorable outcomes on children with immune thrombocytopenia by high dose IV-Ig therapy (Richter, 1995) (Imbach, 1981). Subsequently, IV-Ig treatment was trialed in a variety of other autoimmune disorders. In 1989, Sunakawa reported one of the first cases of beneficial effects of IV-Ig therapy in ocular inflammatory disease. The case described a patient with severe uveitis treated with high-dose corticosteroids, whose visual acuity (VA) was gradually deteriorating. After receiving two courses of IV-Ig, the patient's VA improved, and retinal exudation and phlebitis diminished (Sunakawa, 1989) (Tellier, 2005).

Several mechanisms have been hypothesized for IV-Ig's mode of action. IV-Ig interacts at multiple levels with the immune system, which include the following: (a) blockage and modulation of the expression of IgG Fc fragment receptors on the surface of macrophages; (b) modulation of the activated complement system; (c) modulation of cytokine synthesis and release; (d) modulation of cell proliferation, migration, and apoptosis; (e) modulation of B and T lymphocytes; (f) blockage and modulation of neutrophil cell activation and proliferation; (g) neutralization of circulating autoantibodies; (h) interaction with other B and T lymphocyte surface molecules (Tellier, 2007). The beneficial properties of IV-Ig last beyond the half-life of IgG, providing evidence that the effects are more than a mere passive neutralization of pathogenic autoantibodies (A. Durandy, 2009) (S.V. Kaveri, 2011).

A complete understanding of its role in immunomodulation is yet to be elucidated. Further research into the precise mechanisms of IV-Ig, with an emphasis on autoimmune diseases will eventually lead to a thorough understanding of IV-Ig.

The purpose of this chapter is to highlight the proposed mechanisms of IV-Ig, recognize their beneficial role in the treatment of ocular autoimmune diseases, and emphasize the importance of prioritizing investigations to study the possible, additional benefits IV-Ig has to offer.

Mechanism of Action

Inflammation is designed to be a protective biological response against potentially harmful stimuli. The purpose of an inflammatory response is to remove the initial cause of injury, and avoid consequences of this injury. Autoimmune diseases arise as a result of dysfunctional innate and adaptive immune responses, over-responding to self-antigens, leading to attack on healthy normal self-tissues (Vitale). Although incompletely understood, the following descriptions provide theoretical constructs for the mechanism of action of IV-Ig on each part of the immune system.

B-Lymphocytes

In the event of autoimmune diseases, the stimuli activating B-cells are autoantigens or non-specific polyclonal activation, resulting in production of antibodies against autoantigens. Hindering autoantibodies binding to target autoantigens theoretically may result in alleviation of symptoms seen in antibody-mediated autoimmune diseases (Rajabally, 2009) (S.V. Kaveri, 2011) (A. Durandy, 2009).

IV-Ig impairs B-lymphocyte activity by numerous aspects; the wide panel of anti-idiotypic antibodies, which bind to autoantibodies and interfere with their action against target autoantigens. Other effects include inhibition of antibody production, inhibition of B-lymphocyte differentiation, inhibition of production of interleukin-6 (IL-6) and tumor necrosis factor-α (TNF- α), induction of B-lymphocyte apoptosis, down-regulation of specific auto-reactive B-lymphocytes, regulation of B-lymphocyte subsets expressing CD5, therefore suppressing the auto-antibody producing CD20+ cells, and accelerating breakdown of endogenous IgG (Rajabally, 2009) (A. Durandy, 2009) (S.V. Kaveri, 2011).

T-Lymphocytes

T-lymphocytes are essential players in autoimmunity development, and dysregulation of their function is suggested to trigger pathogenic autoantibody production. In the event of autoimmune diseases, the T-cells are primed to recognize autoantigens (Rajabally, 2009). IV-Ig has been shown to decrease T-cell production of IL-2 and interferon-gamma (IFN-γ), thereby reducing T-cell proliferation and activation. Also, anti-CD4 cells, anti-HLA class I and II, anti-chemokine receptors, anti-CCR-5, and anti-T-cell receptor β chain antibodies are found in IV-Ig preparations, suppressing the development of autoimmunity (L. Padet, 2011) (Rajabally, 2009).

Complement System

In the instance of autoimmune pathology, the membrane attack complex (MAC) is directed towards self-antigens and induces tissue damage (A. Durandy, 2009) (Rajabally, 2009). IV-Ig blunts autoantigen mediated MAC formation, as IV-Ig preparations include anti-C1, C3a, Cb, and C4 antibodies, along with accelerated C3b degradation, resulting in decreased subsequent tissue destruction. The Fc regions of IgG molecules in IV-Ig have the ability to bind to active complement fragments, C3b, C4b, C3a, and C5a, inhibiting immune mediated damage. This complement-scavenging ability is not restricted to a specific Ig phenotype; IgM is more effective than IgG, though IgG is more abundant in IV-Ig preparations (A. Durandy, 2009) (Rajabally, 2009).

Cytokines

Immunomodulating regulators, consisting of a diverse group of proteins and glycoproteins, act as signaling molecules during an immune reaction. The idea of dysregulation of the cytokine system playing a role in autoimmune disorders is under evaluation. IV-Ig inhibits TNF-α mediated cytotoxicity and contains IL-1 receptor antagonists (Rajabally, 2009).

Cell Migration

One of the proposed factors involved in autoimmune diseases is leukocyte migration across biological barriers causing organ specific damage. IV-Ig reduces the expression of intercellular adhesion molecules-1 (ICAM-1), contains anti-integrin antibodies, and inhibits chemokine receptor-5 (CCR-5) (Rajabally, 2009).

Clinical Applications

Currently, IV-Ig therapy is FDA-approved for use in the following extraocular autoimmune diseases: idiopathic thrombocytopenic purpura (ITP), acute myasthenia gravis, dermatomyositis, Guillain Barré syndrome, Kawasaki disease, multi-focal neuropathy with conduction block (MNCB) and chronic inflammatory demyelinating polyneuropathy (Sumru Onal, 2006) (H-P Hartnug, 2009).

Therapeutic Application of IV-Ig

Chronic ocular inflammation, a term that collectively describes a number of heterogeneous autoimmune-mediated diseases of the eye, has a current standard of care involving combinations of corticosteroids, immunomodulatory systemic therapy, and surgical intervention, as applicable to each unique case. Treatment of ocular inflammatory disease should generally be approached in a step-wise fashion, except in case of impending catastrophic damage to structures critical to vision; that is, selection of therapies should focus from least to more aggressive, depending upon clinical presentation, subjective improvement, and always, the mitigation of unfavorable side effects potentially associated with therapy. Corticosteroid treatment, in local, topical, and systemic forms, is over-utilized, regrettably, secondary to ophthalmologists' general lack of understanding of the risk/benefit calculation for corticosteroid-sparing therapy. Immunomodulatory therapies, when employed in the mode of rheumatologic disease therapy, greatly outweigh these risks, given the resultant predictable toxicity of prolonged corticosteroid therapy and loss of vision secondary to delay in implementation of alternative sight-saving therapy. Conventional immunomodulatory agent(s) are useful in controlling inflammation of autoimmune mediated ocular diseases, but efficacy may be limited in severe resistant cases. Therefore, the ability of IV-Ig to efficiently control ocular inflammation with limited side effects and in lieu of chronic corticosteroid use are the most favorable qualities to clinicians.

The following ocular inflammatory diseases represent the indications with the strongest clinical data for IV-Ig use. It is noted that overall, data are scant, as prospective clinical trials in ocular inflammatory disease are limited in size and quantity, derived from the logistical difficulties in mounting randomized controlled trials in rare diseases.

Ocular Cicatricial Pemphigoid

"Cicatricial" in Latin means scar and "pemphigoid" in Greek means blister or swelling. Cicatricial pemphigoid was originally described in the 18th century; onwards, many researchers, clinicians and scientists have been studying this disease in an effort to achieve a deeper understanding of its pathogenesis. Ocular cicatricial pemphigoid (OCP) is an ocular manifestation of a systemic antibody-mediated cytotoxic autoimmune disease, mucous membrane pemphigoid (MMP). Approximately 80% of patients with MMP have ocular involvement. The estimated incidence of OCP is 1 in 20,000 to 1 in 46,000 ophthalmic cases. It is a relatively rare disease, mainly affecting the elderly, with a mean age of onset of 64.5 years, and ranging from 20 to 87 years. Women are more frequently affected than men, with a ratio of 2-3:1, without known propensity towards any particular race or geographic region (Jakobiec, 2011) (Muna Ahmed, 2004).

The pathogenesis of MMP is characterized by autoantibodies (IgG, IgA, IgM) and complement 3 component (C3), binding to an antigen (the beta 4 peptide of alpha 6 beta 4 integrin) in the intracellular portion of hemidesmisomes of the basal epithelial cells of mucus membranes (conjunctiva, oral cavity, nose, pharynx, esophagus, larynx, trachea, genitalia and anus) and less commonly, epidermis (Maza, 2004) (Jakobiec, 2011). Clinical signs and symptoms are dependent on the tissue involved and damage induced at these locations. Ocular cicatricial pemphigoid is the result when conjunctiva is the target, causing chronic conjunctivitis and bullae of mucus membranes, leading to progressive scarring and shrinkage of the conjunctiva (Muna Ahmed, 2004). Progressive cicatrization of the conjunctiva causes vision loss, leading to eventual bilateral blindness consequent to the effects on the cornea of dryness, corneal damage from trichiasis, and from the sandpapering effect of squamous metaplasia of the tarsal conjunctiva of the posterior lid margin. (Maza, 2004) (Muna Ahmed, 2004).

Early diagnosis of OCP is crucial for halting the progression of the disease and prevention of its vision threatening consequences, as any fibrotic damage is irreversible. A combination of clinical findings and immunohistopathology of biopsied conjunctiva leads to diagnosis. (Maza, 2004) (Jakobiec, 2011) (Muna Ahmed, 2004). The rate of biopsy positivity is greatly dependent upon the techniques utilized, the experience of the person performing the biopsy, and of the personnel handling, processing and analyzing the tissue. (Muna Ahmed, 2004).

If diagnosis of OCP is established, it is essential to identify the disease as an ocular manifestation of a systemic autoimmune disease to appropriately select treatment modalities aiming to address the systemic immune dysfunction, and subsequently control the ocular consequences. Adequate arrest of inflammation and prevention of progression is typically achieved with systemic immunomodulatory therapy (Jakobiec, 2011) (Jennifer E. Thorne, 2008).

Treatment of OCP in stage 1 or 2, or with mild to moderate inflammation slowly progressive, involves first line medication such as methotrexate, azathioprine, mycophenolate mofetil or diaminodiphenylsulfone (Jakobiec, 2011) (Maza, 2004). OCP in stage 3 or 4, moderate to severe inflammation or rapidly progressive, requires more aggressive treatment. Combination therapy with cyclophosphamide and short-term use of high dose oral corticosteroids (≥ 40mg/day) is recommended as appropriate management. (Jakobiec, 2011) (Muna Ahmed, 2004) (Jennifer E. Thorne, 2008). Alternatively (and even more effective), combination chemotherapy of rituximab and IV-Ig may be employed, if one can accomplish all that must be accomplished in order for such expensive therapy to be covered by insurance for off-label use.

In 1997, Urcely et al. reported the first application of IV-Ig in two OCP patients unresponsive to corticosteroids and immunosuppressive therapy. Favorable results were identified in both of these patients. (Urcely, 1997) (Tellier, 2005). In a non-comparative, interventional case series, Foster et al. evaluated the effects of IV-Ig treatment in ten patients with biopsy-proven progressive cicatricial pemphigoid with ocular manifestations who previously did not respond adequately to conventional immunomodulatory regimens. IV-Ig was administered at a dosage of 2 to 3g per kg per cycle divided over three days, and repeated every two to six weeks. The duration of therapy ranged from 16 to 23 months (mean, 19.3 months). The optimal therapeutic effect was identified and maintained after a minimum of 4 cycles and maximum of 12 cycles of therapy before disease control. Resolution of extraocular mucosal lesions was observed in nine of the ten patients. Subjective improvement of discomfort and photophobia was reported in all ten patients, and objective improvement or stabilization in visual acuity was established in all patients. The results of this study demonstrated cessation of clinical progression and resolution of chronic conjunctivitis in all ten patients (Ahmed, 1999). A secondary study was conducted by Sami et al. among 15 patients with mucous membrane pemphigoid, of whom 13 had ocular involvement who had failed to respond to high-dose systemic corticosteroids and immunosuppressive agents. All 15 patients received an IV-Ig dose of 1-2g per kg per cycle. All of the patients had an effective clinical response, were able to discontinue previous systemic therapies, and eventually achieved a prolonged clinical remission. No serious side effects were observed (Sami N, 2002). Additionally, Letko et al. conducted a nonrandomized study comparing the clinical outcomes in OCP patients managed with conventional immunosuppressive therapy versus IV-Ig therapy. The results of this study revealed IV-Ig is more effective in arresting progression, controlling inflammation (shorter time between onset of therapy and clinical remission) and preventing recurrences, when compared to patients controlled with conventional immunosuppressive therapy (patients with OCP that were previously resistant to control with conventional agents) (Maza, 2004).

As mentioned above, combination chemotherapy utilizing IV-Ig in conjunction with rituximab has exhibited favorable outcomes in this disease subset as well. Foster et al. conducted a study in six patients with biopsy proven OCP. Prior to this study, four had progressive scarring to the level of legal blindness in one eye; the other two patients had persistent conjunctival inflammation despite aggressive systemic chemotherapy. These six patients were treated with a median of 12 infusions of rituximab over six months, and nine to 41 IV-Ig infusions (median 25.5). The outcome of this study revealed none of the treated patients had progression of scarring, all of the patients maintained their vision in the better eye, and no adverse events were discovered (Maza, 2004). Follow-up data are still being collected on these patients, and are pending publication.

As illustrated from the results of the studies discussed above, IV-Ig is safe and effective therapy for patients with OCP (recalcitrant or otherwise). Proper prescription and employment may result in significant alleviation of symptoms, effective control of inflammation, cessation of progression and prevention of recurrence (Muna Ahmed, 2004). IV-Ig may be the most effective of all therapies described to date for treatment of this disease, especially if combined with rituximab.

Uveitis

Idiopathic

Uveitis, inflammation of any or all components of the uveal tract, is the third leading cause of preventable blindness worldwide; it occurs in patients of all age groups, affecting men and women equally and accounts for 10-15% of all cases of blindness in the United States. Idiopathic uveitis is the most common cause of anterior uveitis (37.8%), intermediate uveitis (69.1%), and panuveitis (22.2%); it is the second most common cause of posterior uveitis (12.3%) and uveitis in children (29%) (Vitale).

Diagnosis of uveitis is not difficult, but assigning a cause for it can be, and when such cause determination is possible, it comes as a result of comprehensive assessment of patient's past medical and family history, review of systems, systemic and ocular examinations, ocular imaging and extensive laboratory workup. Despite rigorous efforts, one in every two cases of uveitis may not have a determinable cause, and are deemed "idiopathic." Idiopathic uveitis is primarily controlled with the use of corticosteroids. However, if inflammation persists in spite of corticosteroid therapy or is recurrent when corticosteroid therapy is discontinued, corticosteroid-sparing immunomodulatory therapy is adamantly recommended as the standard of care. When patients are unresponsive and/or experiencing side effects of conventional immunomodulatory therapy causing dose alteration or discontinuation of the medication, administration of IV-Ig is an appealing alternative (Tellier, 2005) (Sumru Onal, 2006). Ahmed et al. assessed the efficacy of IV-Ig therapy in patients with severe uveitis otherwise unresponsive to conventional immunomodulatory agents. The study consisted of five patients with severe and recalcitrant uveitis. The duration of IV-Ig therapy was 3 to 36 months (mean, 16.8 months). Three of the five patients had intraocular inflammation adequately controlled. In all three of these patients, visual acuity was stabilized or improved. One of three patients with successful response to IV-Ig required maintenance of systemic steroids at a dose of 10 mg per day, while the others successfully tapered systemic corticosteroids. Immediate or long-term adverse side effects were not observed in any of the five patients (Onal S, 2006). In another report, Rosenbaum et al.

conducted a study among ten patients who met the following entry criteria of non-infectious uveitis; active inflammatory disease, and failure to respond adequately to immunosuppressive medication. Initially, two patients with idiopathic uveitis who had previously failed to respond to conventional immunosuppressive therapy were treated with IV-Ig. Encouraging results with regards to abolition of ocular inflammation were observed in one of the patients, leading to an open-label study with eight additional patients. These eight patients were affected with idiopathic intraocular inflammation (3), birdshot retinochoroidopathy (1), sarcoidosis associated anterior and posterior uveitis (1), Behçet's disease (1), scleritis with panuveitis (1), and inflammatory bowel disease with anterior and posterior uveitis (1). Patients were followed for a median of 11 months, and received a median of 7.5 treatment cycles. Five of the ten patients had clinically significant and sustained improvement in visual acuity. Two of the eight patients had markedly reduced their concomitant immunosuppressive therapy.

Onal et al. in a case report, assessed the efficacy of IV-Ig in a 15-year-old male patient with bilateral idiopathic panuveitis who had failed numerous conventional immunomodulatory agents including methotrexate, mycophenolate mofetil, cyclosporine A, cyclophosphamide, and daclizumab. The patient underwent pars plana vitrectomy in both eyes due to significant vitreous pathology. At the time of IV-Ig therapy initiation, VA was declined in the left eye. The initial IV-Ig dose was 1g per kg every 4 weeks. The patient had significant anterior chamber inflammation in the left eye, necessitating an IV-Ig dose increased (to 1.5g per kg every 6 weeks); at the most recent examination, VA improved three lines in the left eye, was maintained in the right eye, and both eyes were free of all inflammation. The patient received a total of 36 months of IV-Ig treatment with complete quiescence, maintenance of excellent VA in both eyes without the requirement of further intervention, and discontinuation of all systemic corticosteroid therapy while on IV-Ig (Onal S, 2006). These studies collectively suggest that IV-Ig therapy may be an effective option in treating patients with uveitis refractory to conventional immunosuppressive therapy.

Birdshot Retinochoroidopathy

Birdshot retinochoroidopathy (BSRC) comprises 6.0-7.9% of cases of posterior uveitis. The onset typically occurs between the ages of 15-79 years, with an average age of 53 years, and presents more frequently in females.

BSRC is detected more commonly among the Caucasian Northern European population, and less commonly among darker pigmented ethnicities.

Although the exact pathogenesis of BSRC has not been identified, particular genetic associations and autoimmune mechanisms have been suggested to play crucial roles. Strong correlation between susceptibility to BSRC and the HLA-A29 phenotype has been observed; individuals with HLA-A29 positivity have 50 to 224 times greater risk of developing BSRC than those without HLA-A29 positivity. Furthermore, T-lymphocyte reactivity to retinal auto-antigens has been observed, partly explaining the pathogenesis of BSRC in HLA-A29 positive individuals, suggesting involvement of immune dysregulation in genetically predisposed individuals with BSRC (Vitale).

BSRC presents with minimal anterior uveitis; vitritis without pars plana exudate; retinal vasculitis specifically involving perifoveal capillaries; and multiple, bilateral, hypopigmented cream colored lesions at the levels of retinal pigment epithelium (RPE) and choroid more commonly inferior or nasal to the optic disc (Vitale).

Diagnosis of BSRC is based on clinical presentation, including complete analysis of general and ophthalmic history, review of systems, and ocular examination, particularly a display of distinctive multifocal hypopigmented lesions on posterior fundus examination. Laboratory and ocular imaging are appropriate measures to initially confirm diagnosis and rule out possible infectious and non-infectious causes before initiating systemic therapy (Vitale).

Treatment is indicated in active BSRC with early and aggressive immunomodulatory therapy (IMT) to adequately control intraocular inflammation and decrease ocular morbidity. Adjunctive therapy with corticosteroids has an effective role in the setting of inflammatory exacerbations and concomitant with management with IMT (Vitale). However, among BSRC patients resistant to conventional IMT, an alternative is IV-Ig therapy (Vitale).

Kazatchkine et al. evaluated the efficacy of IV-Ig in the treatment of BSRC. Eighteen patients with active BSRC were followed prospectively out of a total of 37 patients recorded. Mean age of patients was 51 years (range 29 to 72 years), HLA A29 positivity in 100% of the patients. Efficacy was assessed by measurement of visual acuity, decrease in inflammation and macular edema on fluorescein angiography. Follow-up ranged from 4 month to 5.6 years. Prior to IV-Ig administration, angiography showed retinal vasculitis in 32 patients and cystoid macular edema in 16 patients. After IV-Ig treatment, inflammation on fluorescein angiography improvement was seen in 17 patients (81%), cystoid macular edema decreased in 65% of the cases and visual acuity of 35 out of 66 eyes (53%) improved, 19 out of 66 eyes (29%) remained the same and 12 of 66 eyes (18%) had worsened. In three patients, treatment was discontinued due to side effects. Overall, IV-Ig was tolerated well and side effects were rare (Cassoux N, 2002).

Kazatchkine et al. in an open-label study evaluated the tolerability and efficiency of IV-Ig treatment among eighteen patients (36 eyes) with active BSRC. All of the eighteen patients had symptoms of blurry vision in at least one eye, and met the five diagnostic criteria for BSRC. The mean duration of disease prior to IV-Ig therapy was 30 months. Previous systemic or periocular steroid therapy was stopped at least two months before administration of IV-Ig therapy. IV-Ig was employed as sole therapy, initially at a dose of 1.6 g per kg every four weeks for six months, followed by 1.2 to 1.6 g per kg every six to eight weeks. The mean follow-up was 39 months, ranging between 12 and 53 months. The initial VA was ≤ 20/30 in 26 eyes, 20/25 in five eyes, and 20/20 in five eyes. The final VA was increased by two lines or more in 53.8% of the eyes and decreased in 7.7%. When present, macular edema improved in half of the eyes, as determined by fluorescein angiography. The following side effects were observed: moderate transient arterial hypertension in seven patients, headache in six patients, eczematous lesions six patients, and hyperthermia in four patients (LeHoang P, 2000). These results show that IV-Ig therapy can efficiently and safely control intraocular inflammation among patients with active BSRC previously resistant to conventional IMT.

Retinal Vasculitis

Primary retinal vasculitis (RV) is a rare entity affecting young adults between the ages of 15 and 40 years of age with no strong sex predilection. Most common causes of retinal vasculitis vary in different regions of the world. For example, Adamantiades-Behcet's disease (ABD) is the most common cause of RV in Tunis, found in 53.9% of patients. Secondary retinal vasculitis, as a result of systemic disease, is much more common, seen in ocular inflammatory conditions such as pars planitis, BSRC, sarcoidosis, collagen-vascular autoimmune disorders, malignancy, neurologic conditions and systemic infections. It is classified as a vision-robbing disease characterized by leaky vessels, vascular narrowing or occlusions, perivascular focal creamy-colored cuffs and sheathing, visualized on ophthalmoscope and confirmed with fluorescein angiography (FA) findings (Vitale). Retinal vasculitis diagnosis is dependent on clinical and angiographic findings. Diagnosis is supported by inflammation in the anterior chamber or vitreous and vessel wall staining or leakage visualized on FA (Vitale).

Indications for treatment in RV are CME, severe vitritis affecting vision, retinal ischemia causing areas of capillary drop-out, or capillary destruction around the foveal avascular zone. Even though stringent treatment formulas have not been proposed for RV, the most commonly used first line drugs are corticosteroids. Specifically, oral corticosteroids have shown to be effective anti-inflammatory controllers in RV. However, high dose or chronic use of corticosteroids are not appropriate long-term treatment modalities; rather, IMT should be instituted as soon as possible (Vitale). Among patients unresponsive to conventional IMT, employing IV-Ig therapy is an appropriate treatment option. The use of IV-Ig has shown promising results in treating systemic vasculitis, portrayed by its ability to reduce the incidence of coronary aneurysms in Kawasaki disease when used within 10 days of onset (Vitale).

Onal et al. in a case report assessed the efficacy of IV-Ig in a 26-year-old female with retinal vasculitis affecting both eyes diagnosed in March 2000. Treatment with methotrexate (MTX) dosage up to 37.5mg per week and systemic prednisone had been unsuccessful. Retinal photocoagulation was performed to ischemic areas of the retina in both eyes. After development of neovascularization elsewhere with intravitreal hemorrhage in the right eye, she underwent pars plana vitrectomy and endolaser photocoagulation. In June 2003, she initiated IV-Ig therapy at a dose of 1.8g per kg at a frequency of every 3 weeks, in addition to MTX 10mg per week and oral prednisone 5mg every other day. Six months after initiation of IV-Ig therapy, MTX was discontinued, along with increase in the dose of IV-Ig to 2.5g per kg every 3 weeks. MTX was discontinued not only because of its failure to control intraocular inflammation, but also due to the desire of the patient to conceive. After 14 months, the interval between infusion cycles was prolonged to every 4 weeks, and to every 5 weeks after 25 months of treatment. Her VA was 20/20 in both eyes at the time of IV-Ig therapy initiation and at the last evaluation, VA was maintained in both eyes. After discontinuation of MTX, the patient was able to conceive two pregnancies successfully. Her final treatment regimen was IV-Ig administered at a dose of 2.5g per kg every 5 weeks, prednisone 10mg per day and aspirin 325mg per day. Her last fluorescein angiogram revealed no active retinal vasculitis and she did not require further intervention to control the intraocular inflammation without relapse. The same study group evaluated a 29-year-old with retinal vasculitis unresponsive to mycophenolate mofetil and combination therapy of mycophenolate mofetil and cyclosporine A. Her ocular disease was complicated by background diabetic retinopathy with diabetic maculopathy requiring panretinal photocoagulation and multiple intravitreal triamcinolone acetonide injections in both eyes. Thr patient received 6 infusion cycles of IV-Ig at a dose 1g per kg every 4 weeks for the first 3 infusion cycles. After the initiation of IV-Ig therapy, the dose of mycophenolate mofetil was reduced to 1g per day. When fluorescein angiography revealed active vasculitis, IV-Ig therapy was increased to 2g per kg every 4 weeks for next 3 infusion cycles. Her retinal vasculitis subsided after an increase in the IV-Ig dose, however the patient decided to discontinue cyclosporine A and IV-Ig treatment. The patient had no side effects. Her macular edema persisted during IV-Ig treatment, requiring intravitreal bevacizumab and triamcinolone acetonide injections in both eyes. Her macular edema was complicated with coexistent diabetic maculopathy. This patient was responsive 3 months after IV-Ig dose increase with total quiescence of the retinal vasculitis (Onal S, 2006). IV-Ig is an appropriate alternative therapeutic modality among patients with retinal vasculitis otherwise recalcitrant to the use of conventional immunomodulatory agent(s).

Scleritis

Scleritis, inflammation of the sclera, is a sight threatening condition characterized by severe inflammation and infiltration of the sclera as a result of destruction of scleral components, leading to loss of scleral integrity. Most commonly, scleritis is first seen in the fourth to sixth decades of life, with a peak incidence in the fifth decade. There is a predominance in females, at a ratio of 1.6:1, without predilection to any specific racial groups, and bilaterality in 41% of cases. Scleritis may potentially be an initial manifestation of a systemic disease; most commonly associated diseases are rheumatoid arthritis, systemic lupus erythematous, ankylosing spondylitis, reactive arthritis, Behçet's disease, gout and atopy. Early diagnosis and medical intervention can arrest the inevitable complications of both ocular and systemic processes and improve morbidity and mortality of the disease (Maite Sainz de la Maza, 2012).

Scleritis is classified into anterior and posterior forms. Necrotizing scleritis, type of anterior scleritis, has been reported to have significantly higher associations with decreased vision, anterior uveitis, peripheral ulcerative keratitis and systemic diseases (Maite Sainz de la Maza, 2012). With any type of scleritis, adequate control of inflammation through medical treatment is achieved with systemic NSAID therapy. However, scleritis with additional associated diseases requires more potent anti-inflammatory therapy. Treating individuals with scleritis plus granulomatosis with polyangiitis (nee Wegener's granulomatosis), polyarteritis nodosa, rheumatoid arthritis, or relapsing polychondritis, with isolated NSAID therapy would be wholly inappropriate. Patients with scleritis associated with potentially lethal systemic vasculitis and with necrotizing scleritis should be managed with aggressive immunosuppressive agents (Maite Sainz de la Maza, 2012). When conventional IMT have failed to adequately control inflammation, IV-Ig has shown encouraging results. However, clinical studies evaluating clinical application of IV-Ig among scleritis patients are scant.

Recommended Dosage and Route

The levels of immunoglobulins are measured in all of our potential patients prior to therapy, specifically to determine immunoglobulin-A (IgA) levels. If they are found to be within normal ranges, the patient can proceed with infusions after informed consent is obtained. When IgA deficiency is detected, IV-Ig infusions are contraindicated due to risk of anaphylaxis. Before each subsequent infusion session, high risk blood monitoring is conducted to retrieve alanine aminotransferase (ALT), aspartate aminotransferase (AST), complete blood count (CBC) with differential, blood urea nitrogen (BUN) and creatinine levels. IV-Ig (IV-Ig Gammagard 10%) infusions are typically employed at a dose of 1-2.5g/kg/cycle of treatment, divided over three consecutive days. The rate of infusion is dependent on the patient's general health, heart rate and blood pressure. The number of cycles is determined by the individual disease characteristics, and each infusion cycle is repeated every 2 to 4 weeks. Pre-infusion medication options are (1) diphenhydramine (1mg/kg in children, 50mg IV in adults); (2) methylprednisolone (120 mg IV); (3) acetaminophen (400mg PO in children, 650mg PO in adults), and are administered 30 minutes before starting each infusion. Thorough discussion and explanation of IV-Ig infusion duration with the patient is a key factor ensuring compliance, and treatment success (Sumru Onal, 2006).

Risks, Benefits and Limitations to Therapy

Side Effects of IV-Ig

IV-Ig has a very low profile of major adverse effects. When side effects do occur, they are generally mild. The most commonly observed severe side effects are myocardial infarction and renal failure. IV-Ig's side effects can be divided into three types: immediate side effects, occurring during IV-Ig infusion, which include anaphylactic reactions or less severe reactions such as hypotension or headache; delayed side effects, occurring hours to days after IV-Ig infusion, which include aseptic meningitis; or late side effects, which include transmission of a viral agent. Approximately 36% of patients receiving IV-Ig infusions will experience adverse effects; however these effects are typically mild and transient. Developing side effects during the first treatment cycle increases the risk of side effects during the subsequent IV-Ig infusions (Shoenfeld, 2004). Side effects to IV-Ig can be alleviated with pre- and post-infusion treatment with analgesia, non-steroidal anti-inflammatory drugs or corticosteroids (Sumru Onal, 2006). Administering IV-Ig infusions over multiple days alleviates the potential side effects of volume-overload and vaso-occlusion (Muna Ahmed, 2004). Side effects reported include headache, fever, chills, nausea, fatigue, arthralgia, myalgia, back pain, flushing, bronchospasm, hypertension, aseptic meningitis, acute renal failure, hemolytic anemia, anaphylaxis, and arterial and/or venous thrombotic events.

The following are absolute contraindications to the use of IV-Ig: (1) selective IgA deficiency, (2) severe systemic reaction to intravenous or intramuscular human immunoglobulins (Sumru Onal, 2006). Patients should be screened aggressively prior to initiation of therapy for these syndromes.

Corticosteroid-Sparing Properties

Corticosteroid therapy causes ocular and systemic side effects, regardless of the route of administration. Although systemic complications are most frequent with oral or parenteral routes, the most common systemic adverse effects seen are endocrine (e.g., adrenal insufficiency, Cushing's syndrome, growth failure, menstrual disorders) and neuropsychiatric (e.g., pseudotumor cerebri, insomnia, mood swings, psychosis) complications. The most common ocular complications are development of cataract and secondary glaucoma.

Therefore, IV-Ig is a therapeutic alternative to decrease use or discontinuation of corticosteroids to control intraocular inflammation.

Other Benefits

Conventional immunomodulatory agents utilized in ocular inflammatory diseases are linked with potential side effects such as bone marrow suppression, increased risk of infection, liver and kidney toxicity, gonadal dysfunction and increased risk of malignancies. Amongst immunomodulatory agents, IV-Ig is the only medication, which treats autoimmune diseases without suppressing the immune system. Concerns of fertility and teratogenicity are absent (Sumru Onal, 2006) (Vitale, 2013).

Disadvantages

Cost is a major concern with IV-Ig. Cost of actual medication and administration is estimated to fall between $8,500 to $20,000 per month in the United States (Rosenbaum, 1999). Additionally, IV-Ig infusions are administered at a tedious, continuous rate: 210 to 240 minutes in an ambulatory setting using a belt-worn infusion pump for three days per month. This may pose a significant burden on a patient and their families and/or caregivers.

IV-IG is also a limited resource to the medical community, and is an inappropriate first-line agent. It is extremely costly, and carries the risk of blood-borne infection transmission. As mentioned in each uveitic subset, we underscore that this therapy becomes a viable option only after failure of other available treatments.

CONCLUSION

Exercising the employment of IV-Ig is a valuable approach for a wide array of conventional treatment-resistant ocular autoimmune diseases. Understanding the mechanism of actions of IV-Ig may be imprecise; however the evidence supporting its favorable impact on ocular autoimmune diseases is indisputable. Since IV-Ig application has been among rare eye diseases, clinical evidence thus far has been results from open studies and case reports.

Moving forward, prospective clinical trials among autoimmune ocular inflammatory diseases will provide unprecedented insight into the effectiveness of IV-Ig as treatment modality (Tellier, 2005).

REFERENCES

Ahmed M, Z. G. (2004, November). Ocular cicatricial pemphigoid: pathogenesis, diagnosis and treatment. *Prog Retin Eye Res*, 23(6):579-92.

Ahmed, F. C. (1999). Intravenous Immunoglobulin Therapy for Ocular Cicatricial Pemphigoid. *Uveitis and immunology service*, 2136-2143.

Cassoux N, G.-B. L. (2002, January). Efficacy of intravenous immunoglobulin in the treatment of Birdshot retinochoroiditis. *J Fr Ophthalmology*, 25(1):23-30.

Foster CS, C. P. (2010, May). Combination of rituximab and intravenous immunoglobulin for recalcitrant ocular cicatricial pemphigoid: a preliminary report. *Ophthalmology,* 117(5): 861-9.

Foster CS, S. D. (2004, October). Ocular cicatricial pemphigoid review. *Curr Opin Allergy Clin Immunol.*, 4(5):435-9.

H-P Hartnug, M. L. (2009, December). Clinical applications of intravenous immunoglobulins (IVIg) - beyond immunodeficiencies and neurology. *Clin Ex Immunol*, 158 Suppl 1:23-33.

Jacob S, R. Y. (2009, December). Current Proposed Mechanisms of Action of Intravenous Immunoglobulins in Inflammatory Neuropathies. *Curr Neuropharmacol*, 7(4):337-42.

Kaveri SV, D. G. (1991, November). Intravenous immunoglobulins in the treatment of autoimmune diseases. *Clin Exp Immunol*, 86(2):192-8.

Kaveri SV, K. T. (2009, December). Intravenous immunoglobulins - understanding properties and mechanisms. *Clinc Exp Immunol.,* 158 Suppl 1: 12-13.

Kaveri SV, M. M.-D. (2011, June). Intravenous immunoglobulins in immunodeficiencies: more than mere replacement therapy. *Clin Exp Immunol,* 164 Suppl 2:2-5.

Kirzhner M, J. F. (2011, July-September). Ocular Cicatricial Pemphigoid: A Review of Clinical Features, Immunopathology, Differential Diagnosis, and Current Management. *Semin Ophthalmol*, 26(4-5):270-7.

LeHoang P, C. N. (2000, Marvh). Intravenous immunoglobulin (IVIg) for the treatment of birdshot retinochoroidopathy. *Ocul Immunol Inflamm*, 8(1):49-57.

Maite Sainz de la Maza, J. T. (2012). *The Sclera* (Vol. Second edition). Springer Science + Business Media.

MM, E. (2008, 2008). History of immunoglobulin replacement. *Immunol Allergy Clin North Am*, 28(4):737-64.

Onal S, F. C. (2006, December). Efficacy of intravenous immunoglobulin treatment in refractory uveitis. *Ocul Immunol Inflamm*, 14(6):367-74.

Padet L, S.-A. I. (2011, December). Neutralization of mitrogenic lectins by intravenous immunoglobulin (IVIg) prevents T cell activation: does IVIg really have a direct effect on T cells. *Clin Exp Immunol,* 166(3):352-60.

Palabrica FR, K. S. (2013, October). Adverse events of intravenous immunoglobin infusions: a ten-year retrospective study. *Asia Pac Allergy,* 3(4):249-56.

Richter C, S. A.-K. (1995, July). Treatment of anti-neutrophil cytoplasmic antibody (ANCA)-associated systemic vasculitis with high-dose intravenous immunoglobulin. *Clin Exp Immunool*, 101(1):2-7.

Rosenbaum JT, G. R. (1999, May). The Treatment of Refractory Uveitis with Intravenous Immunoglobulin. *Am J Ophthalmol,* 127(5):545-9.

Sami N, B. K. (2002, January). Intravenous immunoglobulin therapy in patients with multiple mucosal involvement in mucous membrane pemphigoid. *Clin Immunol*, 102(1):59-67.

Shoenfeld Y, K. I. (2004, March). IVIG for autoimmune, fibrosis, and malignant conditions: our experience with 200 patients. *J Clinc Immunol,* 24(2)107-14.

Sunakawa, M. (1989). High-dose intravenous gammaglobulin therapy for uveitis. *Metab Pediatr Syst Ophthalmol*, 12(4);93-5.

Tellier, Z. (2005, December). Intravenous Immunoglobulin in Eye involvement. *Clin Rev Allergy Immunol,* 29(3):295-306.

Tellier, Z. (2007, September). Human Immunoglobulins in Intraocular Inflammation. *Ann N Y Acad Sci*, 1110:337-47.

The Nobel Prize in Physiology or Medicine 1972. (2013). Retrieved from Nobelprize.org: http://www.nobelprize.org/nobel_prizes/medicine/laureates/1972/

Thorne JE, W. F. (2008, December). Treatment of Ocular Mucous Membrane Pemphigoid with Immunosuppresive Drug Therapy. *Ophthalmology*, 115(2):2146-2152.

Urcelay ML, M. A. (1997, September). Cicatricial pemphigoid treated with intravenous immunoglobulin. *Br J Dermatol*, 137(3):477-8.

Vitale, F. C. (2013). *Diagnosis and Treatment of Uveitis.* Jaypee-highlights medical publishers.

In: Plasmapheresis and Intravenous … ISBN: 978-1-63117-916-7
Editor: Rossana Allegro

Chapter 2

COMPLICATIONS OF INTRAVENOUS IMMUNOGLOBULIN THERAPY

Joseph Kahwaji*, MD, MPH, Jua Choi, PharmD, Stanley Jordan, MD and Ashley Vo, PharmD
Comprehensive Transplant Center, Cedars-Sinai Medical Center, Los Angeles, CA, US

ABSTRACT

The administration of intravenous immunoglobulin (IVIG) is generally safe and well tolerated. However, the treatment of autoimmune disorders usually requires high dose therapy (1-2 g/kg) that may result in a greater frequency of side effects and adverse events. These reactions may be generalized or specific to one organ. IVIG preparations differ in their excipients, physical characteristics (liquid versus powder), and chemical composition. The specific IVIG product administered therefore influences the type and severity of adverse reactions observed. The most common side effect is headache. Rarely, headache can be a symptom of aseptic meningitis. Some generalized reactions include fever, pruritus, rash, myalgia, arthralgia, and blood pressure alterations. These side effects can last for a few hours or several days. Thrombotic events, including acute myocardial infarction and stroke, have been reported with hyperosmolar products and may occur during or a few hours after

* Corresponding Author: Joseph Kahwaji, MD MPH. 8635 W. Third Street, Suite 475W, Los Angeles, CA 90048. Email: Kahwajij@cshs.org.

administration. Acute kidney injury as a result of osmotic nephropathy is well recognized after infusion of sucrose containing IVIG products. The rise in creatinine occurs early after treatment and is reversible in most cases. The development of hemolytic anemia is a more recently recognized complication of high dose IVIG therapy. This is associated with non-lyophilized, liquid IVIG preparations which contain higher anti-blood group (A/B) antibody titers. There are also reports of acute kidney injury occurring as a consequence of pigment nephropathy as a consequence of hemolysis after IVIG administration. Lymphopenia and neutropenia may be detected after IVIG infusion. These cytopenias are self-limited and have not been associated with an increased risk of infection. Electrolyte abnormalities are also observed after IVIG therapy. The majority of cases manifest as pseudohyponatremia. However, true hyponatremia has also been reported. These disturbances usually go undetected and resolve without intervention, but can be clinically significant in the setting of renal insufficiency. Infusion reactions can be prevented by pre-medication with acetaminophen, diphenhydramine, and methylprednisolone. Acute kidney injury can be avoided by using non-sucrose containing products. However, these preparations contain higher anti-A/B titers and may result in an increased risk of hemolysis. Splitting the dose of IVIG and slower infusion rates can reduce adverse reactions. Using subcutaneous immune globulin may be effective for preventing some adverse reactions but this has not been effectively evaluated.

INTRODUCTION

The use of intravenous immune globulin (IVIG) since the late 1970s has sparked a great interest in the treatment of a wide range of pathological conditions including rheumatologic, immunologic, obstetric, and oncological diseases. In addition, IVIG is used to modulate anti-HLA antibodies in patients awaiting solid organ transplantation. With its variety of uses, it is crucial to understand the various side effects and adverse reactions associated with IVIG administration. Familiarity with the various formulations and routes of administration are important to minimize potential side effects and adverse events. This chapter aims to provide insight for the healthcare practitioner regarding the most appropriate IVIG product for specific clinical circumstances and the common side effects associated with these products.

IVIG Composition

IVIG is prepared from pooled human plasma obtained from donor centers or source plasma from blood banks. Isolated from plasma, they are treated with multiple viral inactivation steps to ensure IVIG is pathogen-free. Once the immune globulins are filtered they are purified to remove any possible infectious particles. The IVIG preparation process is very complex but the ultimate product yields differences in excipients (inhibitors of IgG aggregation), physical/chemical characteristics (liquid versus powder), stabilizers, osmolarity, and pH [1]. The differences in these ingredients may ultimately increase adverse events in various patient populations. IVIG products vary in osmolarity from 192-1250mOsm/L. Most liquid IVIG formulations are within physiologic osmolarity of 240-440mOsmol/kg. The pH of IVIG preparations ranges from 4.25 to 7.2. There is less formation of immune globulin dimers with lower pH preparations in the presence of certain stabilizers [2].

IVIG products come in liquid or powder (lyophilized) form (Table 1). Liquid formulations of IVIG products come in 5% or 10% solutions. Ten percent volume is ideal for the fluid sensitive patient since less volume is required. For example, 100g of a 10% solution equals one liter of volume compared to 100g of a 5% solution which equals two liters. Powder or lyophilized formulations come in vials with concentrations ranging from 3% to 12%. The osmolality increases from most to least using the diluents saline, D5W, and sterile water, respectively. Sterile water should be used as diluent when reconstituting lyophilized IVIG (e.g., Carimune and Gammagard S/D) to decrease the osmolal load. Reconstitution of the lyophilized powder may take up to one hour. Adequate time for preparation is recommended before administration to the patient. There have been reports of thrombosis in patients who received hyperosmolar IVIG products. The US Food and Drug Administration (FDA) issued a black box warning of thrombosis for IVIG products regardless of administration route highlighting higher risk in patients with advanced age, prolonged immobilization, hypercoagulable conditions, use of estrogens (e.g., oral contraception), indwelling vascular catheters, history of thrombotic events, and history of cardiovascular disorders. Hyperosmolar solutions may increase viscosity in blood vessels (refer to Thrombotic Events section).

Table 1. Commercially Available Immune Globulin Preparations and Formulations

	Conc	Form	Manufacturer	IgA µg/mL	Glucose/ NaCl/ AA stabilizers	Osmolarity (mOsmol/kg)	pH
Gamunex®-C*** 1, 2.5, 5, 10, 20g IV or SC	10%	Liquid	Talecris/Grifols	46	9-11% glycine	258	4-4.5
Gammaked®*** 1, 2.5, 5, 10, 20g IV or SC	10%	Liquid	Kedrion Biopharma	46	9-11% glycine	258	4-4.5
Gammagard® Liquid 1, 2.5, 5, 10, 20, 30g IV only	10%	Liquid	Baxter	37	9-11% glycine	240-300	4.6-5.1
Privigen® IV only	10%	Liquid	CSL Behring	25	L-proline 250mmol/L	240-440	4.6-5
Flebogamma® IV only	5%	Liquid	Grifols	50	D-Sorbitol, PEG ≤3mg/ml	240-370	5-6
Octagam® 1, 2.5, 5, 10, 25g	5%	Liquid	Octapharma	200	Maltose 100mg/ml, NaCl <30mmol/L	310-380	5.1-6
Carimune® 3, 6, 12g vial IV only	Dilute to 3, 6, 9, 12%	Powder	CSL Behring	Trace	Sucrose 1.67g/g protein, NaCl 20mg/g protein	Sterile Water 192 (3%) 384 (6%) 576 (9%) 768 (12%)	6.6±0.2
Gammagard® S/D 2.5, 5, 10g	Dilute to 5%	Powder	Baxter	≤2.2**	(human) Albumin 3mg/ml;	1250 (10%) 636 (5%)	6.8±0.4

	Conc	Form	Manufacturer	IgA µg/mL	Glucose/ NaCl/ AA stabilizers	Osmolarity (mOsmol/kg)	pH
IV only	or 10%				Glycine 22.5mg/ml		
Bivigam® 5 or 10g	10%	Liquid	Biotest Pharmaceuticals	≤200	0.100-0.140M NaCl 0.20-0.29M glycine	Iso-osmolar	4-4.6

* Information obtained from Individual IVIG Package Inserts; All products are preservative free.

** Gammagard S/D powder is safe to use in IgA deficient patients.

*** Gamunex-C and Gammaked subQ route approved for primary humoral immunodeficiency; IV route only for use in idiopathic thrombocytopenic purpura.

Immune globulins are fragile proteins that require stabilizers to prevent aggregation. These stabilizers include glucose analogs (e.g., sorbitol, maltose, and sucrose), sodium chloride, polyethylene glycol, and amino acids (e.g., L-proline). The presence of aggregated immune globulin molecules may predispose patients to the common side effects, which include headache, fever, and flushing [3]. However, the use of these stabilizers may predispose a patient to various adverse events. For example, the presence of sucrose in some IVIG products can increase risk of sucrose-induced osmotic nephropathy associated acute renal failure.

The various extraction and filtration techniques (e.g., ethanol fractionation, ultra-filtration, centrifugation, ion-exchange chromatography, caprylate precipitation) used to pool IgG may still leave trace amounts of other immunoglobulins such as IgA and IgM. Patients who are deficient in IgA may be at risk of anaphylactic reactions with the infusion of IVIG products due to the presence of anti-IgA antibodies [4]. Gammagard S/D powder may be safe for patients with IgA deficiency because of its extremely low level of IgA of ≤2.2 μg/ml (Table 1). In addition there have been some reports of minimal anaphylaxis in IgA deficient patients receiving subcutaneous immune globulins (SCIG) [5].

Table 2. Common IVIG Side Effects (≥ 5%)

Body System	**Common Side Effects Reported (%)**	**Time of Onset**	**Resolution Time**
Cardiovascular/ Circulatory	Hypotension (5), Hypertension (7), Chest pain (5)	During infusion	1 day
Hematologic	Hemolysis (8% - liquid IVIG products), Thrombocytopenia (15)	48-72 hours after	14 days
Gastrointestinal	Nausea/Vomiting (5), Dyspepsia (6)	During Infusion to 1 day after	1-3 day
General	Fever (6.3), Fatigue (6.3), Flu-like symptoms (5), Arthralgia (6.3), Epistaxis (23)	During Infusion	<7 days
Integumentary	Urticarial (10), pruritus (8), Petechiae (21)	During Infusion	1-4 hours
Musculoskeletal	Back pain (6)	During Infusion	<7 days
Neurological	Headache (8)	During Infusion	<3 days
Respiratory	Cough (7), Pharyngitis (5), Rhinitis (13)	1-3 days after	<7 days

* References: Package Insert Gamunex-C, Institution-specific experience [7], [1].

IVIG products have also resulted in positive anti-Hepatitis B core antibody serology testing since IVIG is created by pooling blood from thousands of healthy donors. Serology testing should be done prior to IVIG or 3 months after infusion in order to prevent misinterpretation of positive results. The effect of this passive antibody transfer may be present for up to 3-6 months post infusion [6].

Recommended dosing for IVIG range from monthly infusions of 0.3-0.6g/kg [1] to high doses of 2g/kg with max 140g (>70kg patients) [7]. Patients who are not able to tolerate high volume (>1L), elevated serum creatinine (>1.5mg/dl), and non-O blood type patients should receive a maximum of 1g/kg in a 24 hour period using liquid non-sucrose IVIG products (e.g., Gamunex®-C, Gammaked®). Cost per gram of IVIG based on average wholesale price (AWP) as of February 21st, 2014 in US dollars include: Carimune® at $53/gm and Gamunex® at $77.77/gm.

Table 3. Premedication Regimen

Premedication (30 minutes before)	Treatment Reason
Acetaminophen* 650mg by mouth (maximum 2000mg/day)	Minimize fever related to infusion
Diphenhydramine* 50mg by mouth (maximum 400mg/day)	Minimize itchiness related to infusion
Methylprednisolone* 40mg IV Push	Minimize itchiness, shortness of breath related to infusion

* Additional doses may be given to patient based on symptomatic management.

Common Side Effects of IVIG

Common side effects (≥5% of patients) of IVIG per package insert include headache, fatigue, nausea/vomiting, back pain, abdominal pain, diarrhea, influenza-like illness, and pruritus (Table 2). These side effects may be attributed to the presence of IgG aggregates in the IVIG product or complement activation during infusion. Most of these side effects resolve from three to seven days post-infusion. In general, common side effects after IVIG infusion may be organ specific and are usually mild to moderate. A majority of IVIG induced side effects may be avoided by pre-medicating at least 30 minutes prior to the infusion, slowing the rate of infusion, and splitting high doses over a period of two to five days[8]. Pre-medications include acetaminophen 650mg tablet by mouth, diphenhydramine 50mg tablet by mouth, and methylprednisolone 40mg intravenous (Table 3).

The most common organ-specific IVIG reaction is headache, occurring 5-20% of infusions [9]. Headache can begin during the infusion or within one day post-infusion. Patients may take additional acetaminophen for headaches. The cumulative recommended acetaminophen dose for chronically ill and adult patients with multiple comorbidities is 2000mg oral in a 24-hour period. Rarely, headache may be a symptom of aseptic meningitis. In a case series of patients with Kawasaki disease, four of 384 developed aseptic meningitis [10]. All four developed symptoms within 48 hours of IVIG therapy. Therefore, further evaluation is warranted if headaches do not resolve or are associated with other symptoms of aseptic meningitis.

Table 4. Methods to Reduce Common and Adverse Side Effects

Patient Type	Ideal IVIG Product - Recommendation
Non-O Blood Type*	• Carimune® (If on dialysis) – Can give Carimune over dialysis so net fluid balance is 0. • Gammaked®/Gammunex® – Split dose over 2-3 days at least 24 hours apart to minimize hemolysis
Thrombosis Risk** (e.g., advanced age, prolonged immobilization, hypercoagulable conditions, use of estrogens (e.g., oral contraception), indwelling vascular catheters, history of thrombotic events, and history of cardiovascular disorders	• Avoid Carimune, Privigen (Institution specific thromboses reported) • Recommend Gamunex/Gammaked split dose
Fluid Sensitive	• Split Gamunex/Gammaked • Use 10% solution vs 5%

* References:* [7], ** FDA letter to manufacturers.

The management of common side effects can be directed toward the specific symptom (Table 4). If patients complain of itchiness, additional diphenhydramine may help (maximum dose diphenhydramine 400mg/day). If patients complain of dyspnea, the IVIG infusion rate should be slowed. The recommended initial infusion rate is 1mg/kg/min to a max of 8mg/kg/min. Additional steroid and diphenhydramine may help improve dyspnea. If supportive medications do not help, infusion should be stopped. Also consider splitting doses if the patient has fluid sensitivity (i.e., chronic kidney disease, cardiac disease). Subcutaneous IVIG may help alleviate systemic side effects but may cause temporary mild-moderate local erythema, tenderness, and soreness [11].

ACUTE KIDNEY INJURY

Acute kidney injury is a well-established adverse event following IVIG therapy. The rise in serum creatinine occurs within days of treatment and is reversible in most cases [12, 13]. Kidney injury is a result of osmotic nephropathy related to excipients that render the IVIG preparation hyperosmolar. These primarily include sucrose and other sugar compounds that are used to prevent aggregation of immunoglobulins and stabilize the preparation. A recent review reported the overall risk of osmotic nephropathy to be small with most cases occurring after administration of sucrose or glucose stabilized products [14]. These sugars accumulate in the proximal tubular epithelial cells causing isometric vacuoles that are easily recognizable by histology (figure 2). Maltose and sorbitol based products are less likely to cause osmotic nephropathy since tubular epithelial cells can enzymatically degrade these sugars [14].

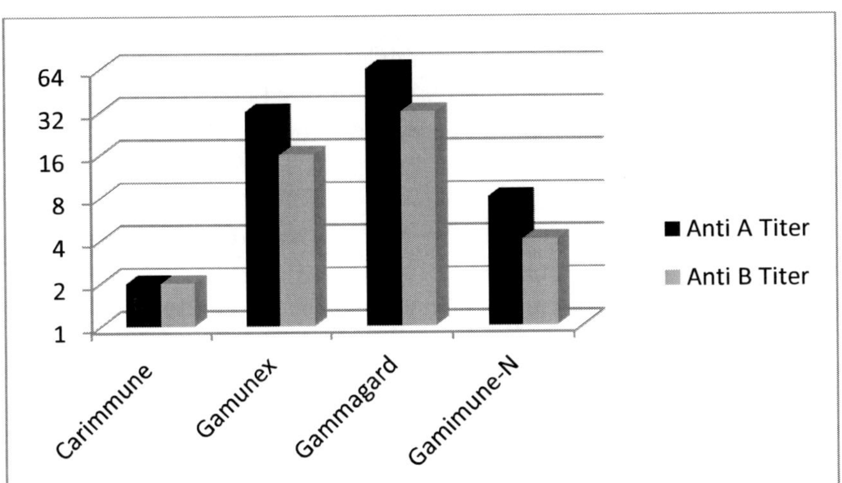

Figure 2. Anti-A and anti-B blood group titers found in different IVIG products. Carimmune, a lyophilized product, had the lowest titers.

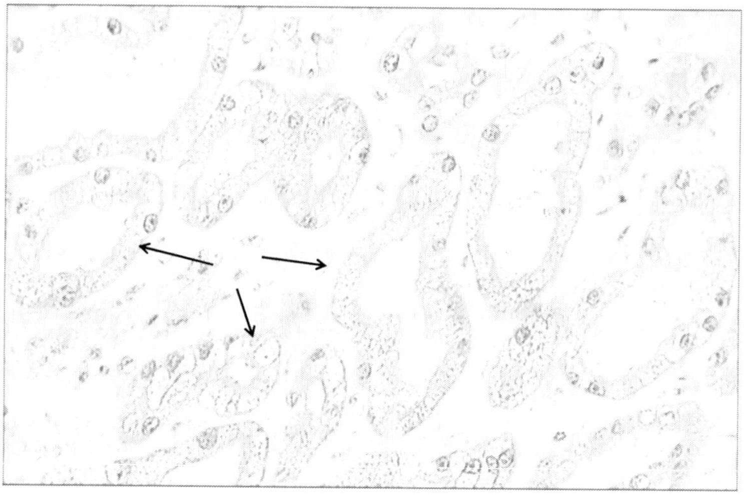

Figure 1. Tubular epithelial cells with extensive isometric vacuolization (arrows) consistent with IVIG induced osmotic nephropathy.
Courtesy of Mark Haas, MD, Dept. of Pathology, Cedars-Sinai Medical Center

IVIG can cause acute kidney injury through other mechanisms as well. There are case reports describing acute kidney injury as a result of pigment-induced nephropathy from hemoglobinuria [15, 16]. Hemoglobinuria results from hemolysis that can occur in non-O blood type patients who receive IVIG products containing high titers of anti-blood group antibodies (refer to *Hemolysis* section). These are typically highly purified, amino acid stabilized products. A case of interstitial nephritis was reported in a patient receiving an IVIG preparation containing mannitol as an excipient. It was thought the use of furosemide contributed to the development of interstitial nephritis in this case [17].

It is important to identify risk factors that increase the likelihood of acute kidney injury after IVIG administration. These risk factors include older age, diabetes, congestive heart failure, and underlying chronic kidney disease as well as other factors (Table 5). A recent case-control study revealed inhibitors of the renin-angiotensin system to be an independent risk factor for IVIG induced osmotic nephropathy [18]. In addition, patients receiving renin-angiotensin blockade had severe renal impairment with 49% requiring temporary dialysis. Those at risk for acute kidney injury may benefit from receiving a sucrose-free IVIG product, maintenance of euvolemia, temporary discontinuation of renin-angiotensin blockade, and close monitoring of kidney function.

Table 5. Risk Factors for Adverse Events following IVIG Administration

Acute Kidney Injury	Hemolytic Anemia	Symptomatic Hyponatremia
Sucrose-based IVIG	Non-O Blood Group	Renal Impairment
Renal Impairment	Liquid IVIG Preparation	SIADH
Elderly	High Dose Administration	Elderly
ACEI/ARB		Osmotically Active Excipients
Volume Depletion		

ACEI = Angiotensin Converting Enzyme Inhibitor, ARB = Angiotensin Receptor Blocker, SIADH = Syndrome of Inappropriate Anti-Diuretic Hormone.

HYPONATREMIA

The most common electrolyte disorder following IVIG administration is pseudohyponatremia. Sodium resides in the plasma water compartment which makes up 93% of plasma. Proteins and lipids compose the non-aqueous phase. IVIG administration increases the non-aqueous portion of plasma and results in a false decrease in the sodium concentration when measured indirectly by ion selective electrodes. This method measures sodium concentration in diluted plasma. Direct ion selective electrodes measure the sodium concentration directly in the plasma water compartment thus eliminating the false low sodium concentration seen in pseudohyponatremia. Steinberger et al. prospectively studied 18 patients receiving IVIG and found evidence of pseudohyponatremia at six and 24 hours after infusion [19]. The fall in sodium concentration correlated with a decrease in the calculated serum osmolality and an increase in the osmolal gap with stability in the measured serum osmolality. Sodium concentration corrected by 10 days post-infusion. The vast majority of patients with pseudohyponatremia remain asymptomatic as it is an artifact of laboratory measurement. However, there has been a report of symptomatic pseudohyponatremia in a 72 year old with multiple sclerosis [20]. The method of sodium measurement was not mentioned in this report. Slowing the rate of subsequent infusions prevented deterioration in this patient's neurologic status. It can be difficult to exclude concomitant true hyponatremia therefore caution is advised if pseudohyponatremia develops in at risk patients (Table 5).

Although rare, true hyponatremia can develop following IVIG administration. It results from osmotically active excipients, namely sucrose, present in IVIG preparations. Sucrose draws water from the intracellular compartment to the aqueous portion of plasma thereby effectively causing a dilutional hyponatremia in those who have impairments in free water excretion. Unlike pseudohyponatremia, dilutional hyponatremia represents a real drop in the plasma sodium concentration that can be symptomatic. Nguyen et al. reported two cases of true hyponatremia after IVIG treatment [21]. One was in a patient with underlying chronic kidney disease stage 5 and another in a patient who developed acute kidney injury after IVIG infusion. True hyponatremia was proven in each case by sodium concentration measurements using a direct ion-selective electrode. The degree of kidney injury in these cases likely contributed to the development of true hyponatremia which has been noted in other studies as well [12].

IVIG preparations are packaged or reconstituted in large volumes of water. This can also contribute to the development of true hyponatremia. Kaneko et al. retrospectively studied 78 patients who received IVIG for Kawasaki disease [22]. Patients with Kawasaki disease frequently have SIADH and therefore are at particular risk of further declines in sodium concentration. Patients were divided into two groups: Group A received IVIG prepared with high sodium concentration (154 meq/L) and Group B received IVIG prepared with minimal sodium concentration (2.6 meq/L). Sodium concentration was statistically lower in Group B attributed to the dilute preparation. The efficacy of the preparations was equal. The authors' concluded that although preparations with high sodium content may be inappropriate for patients with kidney injury or heart disease, it can be considered in children with Kawasaki disease.

Hemolytic Anemia

Acute hemolysis was a previously under-recognized complication of IVIG administration. This complication was non-existent prior to the development of more refined non-lyophilized IVIG preparations. These preparations are derived from the pooled plasma of thousands of individuals and, unlike liquid preparations, have higher titers of anti-blood group antibodies. Varying titers of anti-A/B antibodies in different IVIG preparations were identified with the liquid, isosmolar products having the highest titers (Figure 2). We reported a series of 18 cases of IVIG induced hemolytic anemia in patients with end stage kidney disease receiving IVIG for HLA antibody desensitization [7]. All cases of hemolysis were seen in non-O blood type individuals. In addition, all cases were identified in patients that received high titer formulations and no cases were reported in patients receiving the lyophilized preparations that had low anti-A/B titers. Unfortunately, these low titer products contain sucrose as a stabilizing agent pre-disposing to acute kidney injury and therefore may not be safe for patients with underlying chronic kidney disease or other risk factors for acute kidney injury.

Until recently only case reports and retrospective series describing IVIG-induced hemolytic anemia were reported. Markvardsen et al. published a prospective study evaluating 34 patients who received Privigen (2g/kg) for de novo treatment of chronic neurologic disorders and 50 patients who received maintenance therapy (0.4mg/kg) with either Kiovig or Privigen [23]. They found a significant decrease in hemoglobin associated with a decreased haptoglobin in patients with blood type A or B compared to type O. The development of hemolytic anemia was more pronounced in the de novo, higher dose, group compared to the lower dose maintenance group. The hemolytic anemia was moderate, at worst, in this series.

Monitoring for hemolytic anemia should be instituted for patients considered to be at risk (Table 5). These include non-O blood types, high dose IVIG therapy, administration of high titer formulations, and those with baseline anemia. Common tests helpful in diagnosing hemolysis include a direct anti-globulin test (direct Coomb's), lactate dehydrogenase (LDH), haptoglobin, hemoglobin/hematocrit, and indirect bilirubin. This adverse event can be mitigated by using low-titer, lyophilized products. However, caution is advised in patients at risk for cardiovascular events or kidney injury due to the high osmolality of these products. One approach is to split the dose of IVIG and observe for hemolytic reactions between administrations. Although most cases are mild, symptomatic anemia can occur in patients with underlying anemia prior to the start of IVIG therapy.

THROMBOTIC EVENTS

Thrombotic events are a rare, but concerning adverse effect of IVIG administration. Both arterial and venous thrombosis has been reported in the literature. These events include deep vein thrombosis, pulmonary embolism, myocardial infarction, and stroke. The majority of events occurred within 24 hours of IVIG infusion with close to half occurring within four hours [24]. The most likely mechanism of thrombosis is increased plasma viscosity related to the large amount of protein administered. Steinberger et al. prospectively studied 15 patients administered 2g/kg of IVIG (Sandoglobulin) given over four to five days. Patients were then followed for the development of hyperproteinemia, increased serum viscosity, and pseudohyponatremia as measured 6 and 24 hours after the last infusion [19]. There was a significant increase in total protein and serum viscosity by 24 hours after the infusion with hyperproteinemia being a significant predictor of hyperviscosity. In this study, one patient developed a pulmonary embolism 24 hours after IVIG infusion. Another possible mechanism of post-IVIG hypercoagulability is increased Factor XIa levels noted in some IVIG preparations [25].

Various reports of myocardial infarction after IVIG administration have been published. We reported five (1.8%) cases of acute MI in a series of 279 patients that received IVIG for HLA desensitization or treatment of antibody mediated rejection [26]. The patients that developed MI were between the ages of 34 and 77 and had additional risk factors for coronary artery disease. Symptoms in all patients developed three to 5 hours after IVIG infusion. All patients recovered without long-term effects. The excipient of the IVIG product administered in these cases was a hyperosmolar sodium chloride solution (1250 mOsm/L at 10%). It was determined that this hyperosmolar product resulted in serum hyperviscosity and initiated the thrombotic event. No further events were noted in more than 250 IVIG infusions after switching to non-sodium based solutions with lower osmolality.

Thrombotic events should be rare with subcutaneous IVIG administration due to the low dose and controlled absorption of the preparation. However, a case of cerebral venous and sinus thrombosis was reported in a 20 year old receiving subcutaneous IVIG for common variable immunodeficiency [27]. The patient also had polycystic ovarian syndrome and was taking ethinyl estradiol. The risk of thrombosis was likely increased in this case by the use of oral contraceptives known to predispose to hypercoagulability.

There are currently no established guidelines aimed to prevent thrombotic events after IVIG infusion. Aspirin can inhibit platelet aggregation and can be administered in patients who are at risk for thrombosis or myocardial infarction. Hydration with normal saline may also be helpful for reducing serum viscosity. Finally, avoidance of hyperosmolar solutions in patients with risk factors for thrombosis and myocardial infarction may help prevent some of these serious events.

Leukopenia and Neutropenia

The development of leukopenia and neutropenia is not uncommon after IVIG administration. Fortunately, the degree of leukopenia and neutropenia is mild and has not been associated with an increased risk of infection. Although the mechanism is unclear, it does not appear to be related to bone marrow suppression since the decline in white blood cell count is rapid following administration [28]. Neutropenia defined as an absolute neutrophil count (ANC) less than 1500 mm^3 was seen in 30% of patients in a case series of 16 patients receiving IVIG for various conditions [29]. The nadir ANC was noted to occur two days following infusion with cell counts returning to normal within two weeks. The authors of this series investigated the possibility of anti-neutrophil antibodies existing in pooled immunoglobulin. These antibodies, or other immunologic components, adhere to antigens expressed on leukocytes causing margination and an apparent decrease in the white blood cell count and ANC. Another study examined IVIG-induced neutrophil cytotoxicity. The authors suggested that IVIG contains autoantibodies against specific neutrophil antigens leading to antibody-dependent cell-mediated cytotoxicity [30].

There are no guidelines for monitoring IVIG-induced leukopenia and neutropenia since it is temporary with little clinical significance. However, it may be reasonable to monitor the white blood cell count and differential in patients that are already leukopenic or neutropenic prior to the administration of IVIG. One may consider holding the IVIG infusion or pre-medicating with corticosteroids if there is a concern for infection [28].

Prevention and Management of Adverse Reactions

In summary, the use of IVIG should be tailored to the specific needs of the patient based on fluid requirements, blood type, and existing comorbidities. By customizing the IVIG treatment, adverse reactions and common side effects may be avoided. Fluid sensitive patients should receive a maximum of 1g/kg/day in a 24-hour period or, if on dialysis, may receive IVIG concurrently with dialysis to minimize fluid gain. The non-O blood type patients should receive liquid IVIG preparations in split doses of 1g/kg/day separated by at least by 24 hours. Sucrose stabilized IVIG may prevent the occurrence of hemolysis and can be used in patients at low risk for acute kidney injury. Pre-medication using acetaminophen, diphenhydramine, and steroid may help avoid infusion related reactions and decrease the severity of pyrexia, urticarial, and anaphylactic reactions commonly experienced with infusion of IVIG. In addition, slowing the rate of the infusion may also help avoid infusion related side effects such as shortness of breath, body ache, fever, and itchiness. If patients are at risk of thrombosis, decreasing osmolality load by using sterile water as diluent, slowing the rate of infusion, and distributing infusion over a period of 2-3 days would be beneficial.

REFERENCES

[1] Gürcan HM, Keskin DB, Ahmed AR. Information for healthcare providers on general features of IGIV with emphasis on differences between commercially available products. *Autoimmun Rev.* 2010: 9(8): 553.

[2] Bolli R, Woodtli K, Bärtschi M, Höfferer L, Lerch P. L-Proline reduces IgG dimer content and enhances the stability of intravenous immunoglobulin (IVIG) solutions. *Biologicals.* 2010: 38(1): 150.

[3] Knezevic-Maramica I, Kruskall MS. Intravenous immune globulins: an update for clinicians. *Transfusion.* 2003: 43(10): 1460.

[4] McCluskey DR, Boyd NA. Anaphylaxis with intravenous gammaglobulin. *Lancet.* 1990: 336(8719): 874.

[5] Horn J, Thon V, Bartonkova D, Salzer U, Warnatz K, Schlesier M, et al. Anti-IgA antibodies in common variable immunodeficiency (CVID): diagnostic workup and therapeutic strategy. *Clin Immunol.* 2007: 122(2): 156.

[6] Arnold DM, Crowther MA, Meyer RM, Carruthers J, Ditomasso J, Heddle NM, et al. Misleading hepatitis B test results due to intravenous immunoglobulin administration: implications for a clinical trial of rituximab in immune thrombocytopenia. *Transfusion.* 2010: 50(12): 2577.

[7] Kahwaji J, Barker E, Pepkowitz S, Klapper E, Villicana R, Peng A, et al. Acute hemolysis after high-dose intravenous immunoglobulin therapy in highly HLA sensitized patients. *Clin J Am Soc Nephrol.* 2009: 4(12): 1993.

[8] Katz U, Achiron A, Sherer Y, Shoenfeld Y. Safety of intravenous immunoglobulin (IVIG) therapy. *Autoimmun Rev.* 2007: 6(4): 257.

[9] Bonilla FA. Intravenous immunoglobulin: adverse reactions and management. J Allergy Clin Immunol. 2008: 122(6): 1238.

[10] Kemmotsu Y, Nakayama T, Matsuura H, Saji T. Clinical characteristics of aseptic meningitis induced by intravenous immunoglobulin in patients with Kawasaki disease. *Pediatr Rheumatol Online J.* 2011: 9: 28.

[11] Berger M. Subcutaneous immunoglobulin replacement in primary immunodeficiencies. *Clin Immunol.* 2004: 112(1): 1.

[12] Daphnis E, Stylianou K, Alexandrakis M, Xylouri I, Vardaki E, Stratigis S, et al. Acute renal failure, translocational hyponatremia and hyperkalemia following intravenous immunoglobulin therapy. *Nephron Clin Pract.* 2007: 106(4): c143.

[13] Orbach H, Tishler M, Shoenfeld Y. Intravenous immunoglobulin and the kidney--a two-edged sword. *Semin Arthritis Rheum.* 2004: 34(3): 593.

[14] Dantal J. Intravenous immunoglobulins: in-depth review of excipients and acute kidney injury risk. *Am J Nephrol.* 2013: 38(4): 275.

[15] Ririe MR, Blaylock RC, Morris SE, Jung JY. Intravenous immune globulin therapy for Stevens-Johnson syndrome/toxic epidermal necrolysis complicated by hemolysis leading to pigment nephropathy and hemodialysis. *J Am Acad Dermatol.* 2013: 69(2): 221.

[16] Welles CC, Tambra S, Lafayette RA. Hemoglobinuria and acute kidney injury requiring hemodialysis following intravenous immunoglobulin infusion. *Am J Kidney Dis.* 2010: 55(1): 148.

[17] Tanaka H, Waga S, Tateyama T, Sugimoto K, Kakizaki Y, Yokoyama M. Acute tubulointerstitial nephritis following intravenous immunoglobulin therapy in a male infant with minimal-change nephrotic syndrome. *Tohoku J Exp Med.* 1999: 189(2): 155.

[18] Moulis G, Sailler L, Sommet A, Lapeyre-Mestre M, Montastruc JL, Centers FAoRP. Exposure to inhibitors of the renin-angiotensin system is a major independent risk factor for acute renal failure induced by sucrose-containing intravenous immunoglobulins: a case-control study. *Pharmacoepidemiol Drug Saf.* 2012: 21(3): 314.

[19] Steinberger BA, Ford SM, Coleman TA. Intravenous immunoglobulin therapy results in post-infusional hyperproteinemia, increased serum viscosity, and pseudohyponatremia. *Am J Hematol.* 2003: 73(2): 97.

[20] Bern M. Clinically significant pseudohyponatremia. Am J Hematol. 2006: 81(7): 558.

[21] Nguyen MK, Rastogi A, Kurtz I. True hyponatremia secondary to intravenous immunoglobulin. *Clin Exp Nephrol.* 2006: 10(2): 124.

[22] Kaneko K, Hirabayashi M, Tateiwa A, Shimo T, Teranishi K, Tanaka S, et al. Immunoglobulin preparations affect hyponatremia in Kawasaki disease. *Eur J Pediatr.* 2010: 169(8): 957.

[23] Markvardsen LH, Christiansen I, Harbo T, Jakobsen J. Hemolytic anemia following high dose intravenous immunoglobulin in patients with chronic neurological disorders. *Eur J Neurol.* 2013.

[24] Paran D, Herishanu Y, Elkayam O, Shopin L, Ben-Ami R. Venous and arterial thrombosis following administration of intravenous immunoglobulins. *Blood Coagul Fibrinolysis.* 2005: 16(5): 313.

[25] Wolberg AS, Kon RH, Monroe DM, Hoffman M. Coagulation factor XI is a contaminant in intravenous immunoglobulin preparations. *Am J Hematol.* 2000: 65(1): 30.

[26] Vo AA, Cam V, Toyoda M, Puliyanda DP, Lukovsky M, Bunnapradist S, et al. Safety and adverse events profiles of intravenous gammaglobulin products used for immunomodulation: a single-center experience. *Clin J Am Soc Nephrol.* 2006: 1(4): 844.

[27] Min J, Bhatt A, Aburashed R, Burton S. Cerebral venous and sinus thrombosis associated with subcutaneous immunoglobulin injection and oral contraceptive use. *Neurol Sci.* 2012: 33(3): 627.

[28] Baxley A, Akhtari M. Hematologic toxicities associated with intravenous immunoglobulin therapy. *Int Immunopharmacol.* 2011: 11(11): 1663.

[29] Matsuda M, Hosoda W, Sekijima Y, Hoshi K, Hashimoto T, Itoh S, et al. Neutropenia as a complication of high-dose intravenous immunoglobulin therapy in adult patients with neuroimmunologic disorders. *Clin Neuropharmacol.* 2003: 26(6): 306.

[30] von Gunten S, Schaub A, Vogel M, Stadler BM, Miescher S, Simon HU. Immunologic and functional evidence for anti-Siglec-9 autoantibodies in intravenous immunoglobulin preparations. *Blood.* 2006: 108(13): 4255.

In: Plasmapheresis and Intravenous … ISBN: 978-1-63117-916-7
Editor: Rossana Allegro

Chapter 3

USE OF PLASMA REPLACEMENT THERAPY DURING PREGNANCY

Ernesto González-Mesa[1], PhD,
José M. González-Mesa,[2] MD, Pedro Azumendi-Gómez[1],
Laura Baños Cándenas,[1] MD,
María José Benítez-Marín[1], Ana Guzmán-León[1], MD,
Aurelia Marsac[1], MD and José Herrera-Peral[1], PhD
[1]Department of Obstetrics and Gynecology.
University of Málaga, Málaga, Andalusia, Spain
[2]Department of Anesthesiology. Málaga University Hospital,
Málaga, Andalusia, Spain

ABSTRACT

In this chapter we will review the diseases that most often require the use of plasma exchange therapy during pregnancy. It is well known the important role of plasmapheresis in the removal of the F-VIII multimers observed in the thrombotic thrombocytopenic purpura, but also the auto-antibodies that appear in autoimmune diseases like Myasthenia Gravis, Antiphospholipid Syndrome or Systemic Lupus Erythematosus. There are also some situations where plasma exchange therapy is being used recently with success like Isoinmunization, Gestational Penphigoid, Prymary Hypertriglyceridemia or Acute gravidic liver steatosis.

Throughout this chapter we review the most important clinical and therapeutic features of these illness during pregnancy.

ABBREVIATIONS

AGLS:	Acute gravidic liver steatosis
AP:	Acute pancreatitis
APS:	Antiphospholipid syndrome
ASFA:	American Society for Apheresis
CAPS:	Catastrophic antiphospholipid syndrome
CRP:	C-reactive protein
DALI:	Direct Adsorption of Lipoproteins
FFP:	Fresh frozen plasma
GP:	Gestational pemphigoid
HAS:	Human albumin solution
HTG:	Hypertriglyceridemia
IUGR:	Intrauterine growth restriction
MCA-SV:	Maximum (systolic) velocity of the Middle Cerebral artery
MG:	Myastenia Gravis
NL:	Neonatal lupus
PEX:	Plasma Exchange
PHTG:	Pancreatitis secondary to hypertriglyceridemia
PRT:	Plasma Replacement Therapy
PTE:	Pulmonary thromboembolism
SLE:	Systemic Lupus erythematosus
TTP:	Thrombotic Thrombocytopenic Purpura
USS:	Upshaw-Schulman syndrome

INTRODUCTION

Plasmapheresis is a therapeutic tool used to treat a wide range of disease processes, and in which the priority aim is to ensure sufficient plasma exchange to reduce or eliminate symptoms resulting from the action of pathogenic elements vehiculized in the plasma. Scientific selective apheresis with principles of evidence-based medicine involves the application of one of the oldest therapeutic modalities (bleeding), widely used between the fourth century B.C. and the second industrial revolution. The first publication in the field of apheresis was made by Abel in 1914, though it was not until 1960, with the contributions of Schwab and Frahey, that the benefits of plasma exchange in Waldenström's disease were documented. In 1969 the practice was first applied in obstetrics, specifically in pregnant women with perinatal hemolytic disease. One year later, in 1970, its use was extended to other diseases.

With the consolidation of this therapeutic technique, its indications have increased in obstetrics, and although it is not recommended on a routine basis, plasmapheresis has been used for the treatment of a number of disorders characterized by the presence of circulating antibodies, such as antiphospholipid antibody syndrome, systemic lupus erythematosus, myasthenia gravis, pemphigoid, or thrombotic microangiopathic disorders such as thrombotic thrombocytopenic purpura. Likewise, the technique has been used in situations characterized by multiorgan damage associated with the presence of circulating toxic agents, as in pancreatitis or cholestasis [1, 2]. In order to be able to apply this treatment with the required efficacy and safety, thorough knowledge is needed of the repercussions of apheresis upon the constituents of normal plasma, the role of fluid exchange, and the potential risks associated with the technique.

Plasmapheresis as a therapeutic tool fundamentally involves passing the patient blood through an extracorporeal circuit to separate and eliminate those harmful elements that cause or perpetuate a concrete disease condition, thereby contributing to its treatment [3] (Table 1).

Table 1. Mechanism of action of plasmapheresis

Reduction of specific factors associated with the disease
Immunoglobulins, cryoglobulins, immune complexes, lipoproteins, cytokines
Replacement of deficient factors
Plasma replacement with coagulation factors
Modulation of immune response

The current apheretic procedures with therapeutic intent include the following:

- *Hemapheresis.* This technique separates one or more blood components, and the rest is returned to the patient.
- *Hemoadsorption* (HADS). This technique eliminates a given substance from the blood through an adsorption mechanism.

- *Plasma-adsorption.* This technique is used to eliminate a given substance present in plasma filtered through an uncoated activated charcoal cartridge and an anion exchange resin column.
- *Other methods* in turn are used for the treatment of hyperlipoproteinemias (LDL apheresis, DALI apheresis) to separate substances according to their molecular weight, or specifically for hematological and transfusion therapy.

The following techniques are of particular interest in application to *critical obstetric conditions:*

1. *Plasmapheresis.* This technique separates and eliminates plasma from the rest of the blood components, without replacement.
2. *Plasma exchange.* This technique separates and eliminates plasma from the rest of the blood components, followed by replacement in 1:1 proportion with 5% albumin or fresh frozen plasma.

The benefit of plasmapheresis is based on the rapid depletion of factors associated with the background disease, with the replacement of factors that are deficient in plasma, and the modulation of T cell mediated immunity, inclining the T_{h1}/T_{h2} balance in favor of T_{h2} cells and suppressing the production of IL-2 and IFN-γ [4, 5].

It should be remembered that immunoglobulins have a half-life of 5-21 days, with a vascular distribution consisting of IgG 45% and IgM 75%. This implies that plasmapheresis [6] can eliminate them from the bloodstream. According to the above, the exchange of a plasma volume results in the removal of 45-75% of the circulating immunoglobulins, and larger volume exchanges result in the elimination of much lesser proportions of immunoglobulins; consequently, removals in excess of two plasma volumes are not advised. Following the procedure, macromolecules reappear in the intravascular compartment as a result of lymphatic drainage and simple diffusion through the blood capillaries. The inter-compartmental balancing rate (from the extravascular to the intravascular compartment) is 1-2% after one hour. Five plasmapheresis sessions therefore would be needed to reduce the total systemic immunoglobulins to less than 10% in an interval of 7-10 days.

Likewise, the type of antibody to be removed conditions the frequency and duration of treatment. The half-life of each immunoglobulin differs, ranging from 21 days for IgG to 5 days in the case of IgM. More frequent plasmapheresis sessions are needed to remove IgG, for although its half-life is comparatively longer, only 45% is present in the intravascular space. In turn, frequent plasmapheresis sessions are also needed to remove IgM, for even though 75% of the total is exchanged, the half-life is very short [7].

Substance elimination from plasma can be expressed using the following equation: Y/Y_0= In this expression, Y is the end concentration of a given substance, Y_0 is the initial concentration, and x is the number of times volemia is exchanged during the procedure.

Adequate prescription of the technique requires an estimate of the plasma volume. In this context, normograms are used, based on biometric parameters and the hematocrit. A useful empirical method is to consider a plasma volume of approximately 35-40 ml/ kg, applying the lower limit for patients with normal hematocrit values, and the upper limit in cases of anemia. Kaplan recommends a simplified method for predicting the estimated plasma volume (EPV):

EPV (liters) = 0.065 x weight (kg) x (1 – hematocrit (%)/100) [8]

Technical Considerations and Types of Plasmapheresis [8]

The methods used to perform plasmapheresis comprise centrifugation and transmembrane filtration.

- *Centrifugation* is commonly used in blood banks to separate plasma from the different cell fractions, allowing cytapheresis.
- *Transmembrane filtration* is the method of choice for the treatment of acute obstetric conditions. It is based on the use of high-permeability membranes (large pore size: 0.3-0.6 μm) that allow plasma filtration, retaining only the cellular components. This technique requires a central venous access and anticoagulation with heparin. It does not allow cytapheresis.

The extracorporeal system consists of an arterial line carrying blood to the filter and a return system or venous or afferent line transporting the cellular components and exchange solution back to the patient. This technique requires a specific monitor, which is often that used in hemodialysis. A roller-type pump is needed, allowing blood extraction at a necessary minimum flow rate (150 ml/minute).

Technical Considerations

Vascular Access

Although other vascular accesses such as peripheral veins, accessible arteries or arteriovenous fistulas may be used in concrete situations, the treatment of obstetric critical patients normally involves a central access with temporal catheters providing a minimum flow rate of 100 ml/ minute. The most common complications of these catheters are malpositioning, obstruction and infection.

Anticoagulation

The extracorporeal circuit must be anticoagulated with heparin. Specifically, at the start of each session we administer 0.5-1 mg/kg of 1% heparin sodium, which suffices to cover an entire session lasting 2.5-3 hours. In situations with a high bleeding risk, the starting dose should be reduced, provided the extraction flow rate is adequate. Before starting the session, a basic coagulation study and platelet count are required.

Replacement Solution

The replacement fluid should contain albumin, which is the main determinant of oncotic pressure. Replacement of an equivalent volume with 5% albumin is sufficient. The fluids used are human albumin solution and fresh frozen plasma.

Although fresh frozen plasma is the ideal replacement solution, the risk of anaphylactoid reactions and citrate toxicity, blood group dependency (which limits availability), and the possibility of viral disease transmission, make replacement with albumin solution more advisable.

Human Albumin Solution (HAS)

Human albumin solution at a concentration of 5% contains no preservatives and is characterized by sodium and potassium concentrations of 145 ± 15 and 2 mEq/l, respectively. In certain circumstances, these levels may produce hypopotassemia.

When HAS is used as replacing fluid after a plasmapheresis session, coagulation factor depletion occurs, the prothrombin time may be prolonged 30%, and the activated partial thromboplastin time can increase to double the normal value – followed by a return to normal within approximately four hours. After several weekly sessions, recovery is slower. This makes it necessary to use fresh frozen plasma in patients with defective hemostasis.

HAS is associated with immunoglobulin and complement depletion, which can result in a high risk of infection. In patients with a particularly high infection risk, 100-400 IU/kg of immunoglobulins are administered via the intravenous route after each plasmapheresis session.

Complications [9]

Therapeutic apheresis is quite safe. The incidence of serious complications ranges from 0.0255-0.2% and includes serious anaphylactic reactions related to use of fresh frozen plasma. The associated mortality rate is 0.05%, but most deaths are attributable to the serious background disorders treated with this technique.

Complications Derived from the Replacement Fluids

The use of fresh frozen plasma can cause anaphylactic reactions, with an incidence of 0.2%.

Electrolyte Alterations

The administration of intravenous calcium at the start and end of the session is useful for preventing hypocalcemia secondary to the loss of free calcium retained in the filters, or the loss of calcium bound to albumin.

Infectious Complications

Such infections are exceptional (incidence < 0.5%), but can be favored by immunoglobulin and complement depletion.

Coagulation Alterations and Other Hematological Disorders

Following a plasmapheresis session, most coagulation factors, fibrinogen and antithrombin III decrease 60%. After 24 hours, the fibrinogen and antithrombin III levels reach 50% and 85% with respect to baseline, respectively. The use of fresh frozen plasma for replacement is recommended in patients requiring 3-5 treatment sessions. This can be very useful particularly in patients who may need surgery or are in the immediate postoperative period, as well as in obstetric patients who may have to end pregnancy through cesarean section.

A post-treatment drop in hematocrit is exceptional. The hematocrit may decrease 10% after treatment, due to hemodilution. In patients requiring chronic treatment, sideremia and ferritin levels must be monitored.

Hemodynamic Consequences

The incidence of hypotension is 1.7%. It may occur due to different reasons, such as inadequate replacement volume, vasovagal episodes, anaphylactic reactions and cardiac arrhythmias.

THROMBOTIC THROMBOCYTOPENIC PURPURA

Thrombotic thrombocytopenic purpura (TTP) is one of the microangiopathic disorders that can be diagnosed during pregnancy. These alterations are characterized by the formation of microthrombi in small vessels, leading to thrombocytopenia, microangiopathic hemolytic anemia, and multiorgan damage. Microangiopathic disorders include three entities: TTP, hemolytic-uremic syndrome (HUS) and preeclampsia-HELLP syndrome.

TTP is clinically characterized by a group of 5 symptoms: thrombocytopenia, microangiopathic hemolytic anemia, fever, neurological alterations and renal failure. It can exhibit a familial trait, though idiopathic TTP is the most common presentation. HUS in turn is characterized by renal failure, and although it is typically observed in children with a history of infection due to toxin-producing bacteria in the previous days or weeks, the disease occasionally has also been reported during pregnancy. On the other hand, both preeclampsia and HELLP syndrome belong to a range of disorders in which arterial hypertension is the fundamental clinical feature - HELLP syndrome being one of the most serious conditions.

Epidemiology and Presentations

The reported incidence [10] of TTP in the general population is 3.8 cases per million individuals. In turn, the incidence of TTP and HUS, as disorders differentiated on the basis of laboratory test criteria, is one case in every 25,000 pregnancies [11] and one case in every 198,000 pregnancies [12], respectively.

TTP is more common in women, with a peak incidence in the fourth decade of life, and 10% of all cases occur during pregnancy [13]. The incidence of TTP shows a female/male ratio of 3:2, possibly because of the greater female susceptibility towards autoimmune disorders. Pregnancy triggers both the appearance of the disease and its recurrence [14]. TTP associated to pregnancy accounts for 10-30% of all cases of TTP diagnosed in adults [15, 16].

TTP can manifest in three clinical forms. A first form is familial-hereditary congenital disease or Upshaw-Schulman syndrome (USS), which accounts for a mere 5% of all cases in the general population and 24% of all cases associated with pregnancy [3], while a second form is acquired idiopathic disease (the most frequent presentation), and a third form is related to the use of drugs, infections, neoplasms and pregnancy. The disease often evolves in the form of outbreaks. In this sense, following remission of the initial episode, recurrences of the clinical symptoms are typically observed, particularly during the first year after the diagnosis [17].

In the absence of adequate diagnosis and treatment, the maternal and fetal mortality rates approach 90% [18]. On the other hand, unlike as occurs in HELLP syndrome or severe preeclampsia, there is no evidence that uterine evacuation solves the problem [19]; a correct differential diagnosis is therefore of crucial importance.

Thrombotic thrombocytopenic purpura as either an initial episode or recurrence can manifest at any time during pregnancy [20] though the condition is more often diagnosed in advanced gestation, during the second or third trimester, in peripartum, or even in the puerperal period [21, 22].

TTP was first described in 1924 by Moschovitz in a 16-year-old [23] girl who developed hemolytic anemia, thrombocytopenia, neurological alterations and impaired renal function, followed by death due to cerebral infarction and heart failure. The autopsy revealed generalized thrombosis, particularly of the terminal arterioles. The first documented case of TTP during pregnancy was reported in 1955, in a 30-year-old woman in the eighth month of pregnancy [24], who died as a result of the disease.

Physiopathology

Von Willebrand factor is a multimeric glycoprotein fundamentally produced in the endothelial cells, where it accumulates in the Weibel-Palade bodies, and in megakaryocytes, conforming the so-called alpha granules. These intracellular Von Willebrand factor multimers are larger (ultra-large multimers) than those that circulate freely in plasma under normal conditions (large multimers). The ultra-large multimers are able to bind with greater affinity than the large multimers to the platelet GPIb receptors, thereby favoring platelet aggregation. Regulation of multimer size is therefore essential in order to maintain adequate function.

Regulation of multimer size is mediated by a metalloproteinase known as ADAMTS-13 (A desintegrin and metalloproteinase with a thrombospondin type 1 motif, member 13) that cleaves the ultra-large multimers as they are secreted, converting them into chains that are anchored in the collagen of the vascular wall or circulate freely [25].

Defects in degradation of the ultra-large Von Willebrand factor multimers give rise to the different forms of TTP. The existence of ultra-large Von Willebrand factor multimers in the plasma of patients with recurrent TTP was reported in 1982. These multimers would increase platelet adherence to the endothelium, particularly in high-flow vessels (capillaries), thereby favoring the appearance of thrombi [26, 27].

In the familial forms of the disease (USS), homozygous mutation of the gene encoding for the synthesis of ADAMTS-13 (chromosome 9) causes the protease activity to drop to below 5% of that seen under normal conditions [28]. The familial form usually begins to manifest during childhood, though in some cases it develops later in life, and occasionally during pregnancy. Many mutations have been identified in relation to ADAMTS-13 deficiency, with variable impact in relation to the clinical severity of the condition. Approximately 90% of all patients with both homo- and heterozygous mutations present symptomatic TTP [29, 30].

In the acquired forms, protease activity is low or inexistent during the disease outbreaks, and recovers in the disease-free intervals. In such cases, the existence of an IgG autoantibody targeted to ADAMTS-13 has been identified. Autoantibody production may be transient and/or recurrent, thereby marking the course of acquired idiopathic TTP. Autoantibodies can be detected in approximately 31-38% of all patients with idiopathic TTP.

A significant observation is the fact that all patients with USS who do not receive prophylactic treatment initially develop the disease or experience recurrences during pregnancy, and an important percentage suffer their first episode upon becoming pregnant. On the other hand, 25% of all patients with acquired TTP develop recurrences during pregnancy or in the immediate puerperal period.

Despite knowledge of the mentioned physiopathological aspects of the disease, doubts remain regarding the existence of still unknown additional etiopathogenic factors. The fact that there have been reports of cases of acquired idiopathic TTP in which the ADAMTS-13 levels are normal, or of familial TTP characterized by a complete absence of ADAMTS-13 without clinical manifestations until adult age, points to the need for further investigation of the pathogenesis of this disease [31]. Quantification of ADAMTS-13 in the disease-free intervals contributes to distinguish among the different forms of the disease. In this sense, values of under 10% of normal are typical of hereditary TTP, while values above 30% are indicative of acquired TTP [3].

Treatment

The initial treatment of TTP-HUS during pregnancy is no different from that indicated in the non-pregnant patient [32]. Patients with USS benefit from prophylactic treatment with fresh plasma infusions every 2-3 weeks, according to the ADAMTS-13 [33] activity levels.

TTP is potentially fatal, with a mortality rate of over 90% before introduction of the current treatments. The prognosis, in terms of maternal-fetal survival rates, has improved since the 1970s with the development of treatments such as plasma transfusions and plasmapheresis. The mortality rate has dropped to approximately 10-20%, with a response in up to 90% of all cases of TTP, and healing rates of up to 80%. Plasmapheresis is the most effective treatment option and should be started as soon as possible. Even when the diagnosis is uncertain, the possible complications of TTP outweigh the risks of such treatment [34, 35]. Plasma administration while plasmapheresis is started may be useful [36]. In fact, when plasma exchange cannot be started immediately, it is advisable to start the infusion of high fresh plasma doses under constant central venous pressure control in order to avoid volume overload [37]. Pregnancy does not appear to modify treatment response, though the effects upon the fetus have not been evaluated.

Plasmapheresis is able to eliminate circulating anti-ADAMTS-13 autoantibodies and ultra-large Von Willebrand factor multimers from plasma. The infusion of fresh plasma in turn helps restore the deficient ADAMTS-13 levels. A schematic representation of treatment for acute TTP episodes is provided in Figure 1.

Corticosteroids have some effect in the treatment of TTP episodes. Before the generalized use of plasma exchange therapy, some authors reported a favorable response in 55% of the patients with neurological disorders when using high dose corticosteroids [38]. Subsequent studies have shown the benefit of high dose corticosteroids as adjuvant therapy (dexamethasone 10 mg/kg/day for 3 days and 2.5 mg/kg/day thereafter) [39].

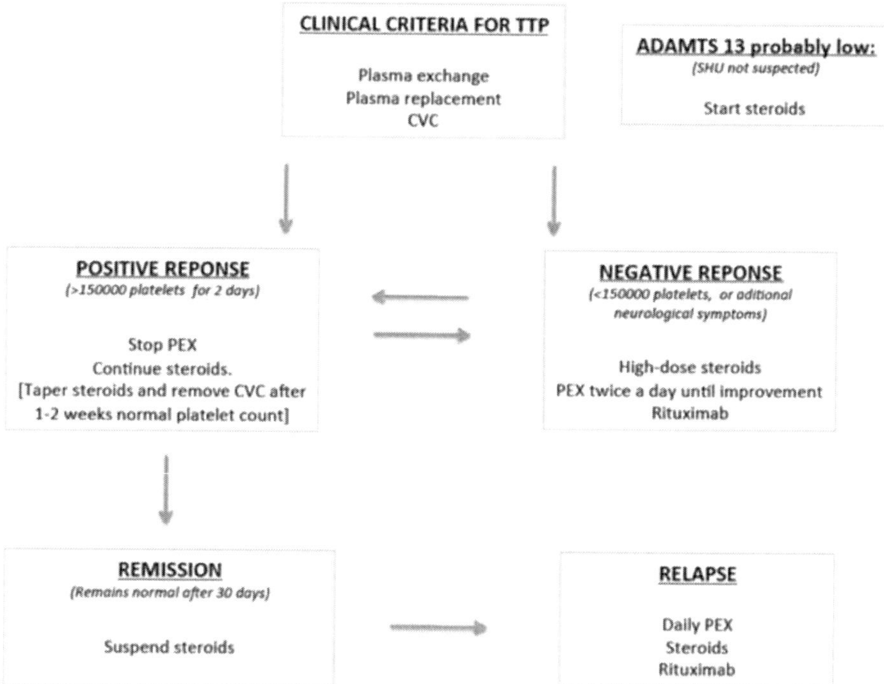

Figure 1. Treatment protocol for TTP patients. Adapted from George JN. How I treat patients with thrombocytopenic purpura: 2010. Blood 2010; 116:4060-4069. *PEX*: Plasma exchange. *CVC*: Central venous catheter.

Although antiplatelet treatment could seem adequate from the physiopathological perspective, some studies have found it to increase bleeding risk. The administration of antiplatelet drugs is therefore not generalized [46]. Nevertheless, some recent clinical guides suggest the administration of 75 mg/day of aspirin or low molecular weight heparin at prophylactic doses, if the platelet count is over 50.000/mm^3 [40].

Platelet transfusion should be reserved for patients with life-threatening bleeding problems, since the worsened clinical condition reported by different authors after platelet transfusion suggests that it worsens the microangiopathic disorder [47]. If platelet transfusion proves necessary, it should always be associated to plasma replacement therapy [46, 41].

In patients refractory to treatment (10-20% of all cases), and when exacerbations of the acute episode occur in under 30 days after normalization of the platelet count, a monoclonal antibody (rituximab) has been shown to be effective as second-line treatment [42]. An 88% success rate has been reported with the administration of rituximab in refractory cases [43]. This monoclonal antibody allows faster platelet recovery, decreases the circulating autoantibody titers, and increases the levels of ADAMTS-13 activity [44]. Rituximab is able to normalize platelet count within an average of two weeks, with disease remission in 5 weeks, and is effective in preventing relapse in the year following treatment. The use of rituximab during pregnancy has been associated with neonatal neutropenia, though it has been administered in the first three months of pregnancy without neonatal adverse effects [45].

Although some studies have reported benefits with other drugs, randomized studies are needed to clarify the role of agents such as vincristine, cyclophosphamide or immunoglobulins via the intravenous route in the treatment of TTP in pregnancy.

Before the introduction of plasma exchange, maternal survival in cases of TTP related to pregnancy was very limited, with a mortality rate of over 90%. However, following the introduction of this treatment modality, the maternal mortality rate has dropped to 0-10% (Figure 1). At present, morbidity remains high, with neurological damage in up to 10% of all cases and renal damage in 21% [46, 47]. In some series the perinatal mortality rate reaches 80% [3. 48], and is usually related to hypoxia due to placental vascular lesions secondary to thrombotic occlusion of the decidual arterioles. No cases of idiopathic TTP in newborn infants have been reported.

Since treatment with plasmapheresis must be started within the first 24-48 hours after the onset of symptoms, any delay in establishing the diagnosis has negative consequences. An adequate differential diagnosis must be established between TTP and HELLP syndrome, since the treatment in each case differs, and confusing the two diseases has been associated to increased maternal mortality [49, 50]. The ending of pregnancy does not improve the course of TTP. It therefore should only be performed when there is evidence of fetal distress or growth retardation, concurrent preeclampsia, or in cases where plasma exchange proves ineffective. Perimortem cesarean delivery has been described in patients with TTP following irreversible cardiorespiratory arrest [51].

The general recommendation for controlling pregnancies of this kind is to closely monitor the patients during pregnancy and start prophylactic plasmapheresis every two weeks if the ADAMTS-13 activity falls to under 10% or blood smears yield unequivocal evidence of red cell fragmentation (schistocytes), suggesting the presence of hemolytic anemia [41]. Plasmapheresis is recommended before delivery.

Myasthenia Gravis

Myasthenia gravis (MG) is a neuromuscular disease of autoimmune origin that affects the skeletal muscle and is characterized by the presence of antibodies targeted to the nicotinic acetylcholine receptors of the motor end plate – a condition that prevents nerve impulse transmission and causes weakness and fatigability. The antibodies block the acetylcholine receptors, which undergo endocytosis and subsequent destruction, with activation of the complement deposit in the postsynaptic membrane. Patients with MG often present other autoimmune disorders such as hypothyroidism, rheumatoid arthritis, pernicious anemia, vitiligo, polymyositis and systemic lupus erythematosus.

Although MG may occur at any age, it is more common in women in their thirties. On the other hand, a series of factors are known to favor the development of severe muscle weakness episodes, including particularly the use of relaxants and anesthetics, intercurrent infections, menstruation, anxiety, pregnancy and puerperium [52].

Pregnancy can trigger the onset of the disease in previously asymptomatic patients, or exacerbate it in patients who already have MG. Any course of the disease is possible, however: exacerbation, myasthenic attacks, or total or partial remission - an important prognostic factor being the disease status before pregnancy. Thirty percent of all patients with MG worsen when becoming pregnant, particularly during the first trimester [53].

The diagnosis is suspected from the clinical manifestations, which are characterized by muscle weakness, initially affecting the extrinsic muscles of the eye, with the frequent occurrence of diplopia and palpebral ptosis. Involvement of the other cranial muscles usually precedes weakness in the lower and upper extremities, with improvement after rest. Although affected patients suffer permanent muscle weakness, more evident at the end of the day, the development of a severe attack may prove life-threatening due to paralysis of the respiratory muscles [54].

A number of techniques such as electromyography or the Tensilon test (administration of edrophonium, a short-acting acetylcholine esterase inhibitor that notoriously improves muscle weakness) can help confirm the diagnosis. On the other hand, antibodies targeted to the acetylcholine receptor (AChR) are present in 80% of all patients with generalized weakness and in 50% of those with ocular manifestations. It has been observed that 70% of all seronegative patients have antibodies against muscle receptor-specific tyrosine kinase [55], and 9% have antibodies against lipoprotein receptor-related protein 4 of the motor [56] end plate - these findings indicating the existence of more than one underlying physiopathological mechanism.

Up to 80% of all pregnant women with MG can present thymus gland hyperplasia, and 10% of all myasthenic women over 30 years of age develop thymomas requiring surgical treatment.

Treatment of patients with MG during pregnancy should be individualized, depending on the degree of muscle weakness and respiratory muscle involvement. Thymectomy is not indicated during pregnancy, though it should be considered during preconception counseling in patients with marked thymus gland hyperplasia and symptoms. In mild cases, the use of cholinesterase inhibitors such as pyridostigmine (30-60 mg administered 3-4 times a day) may be sufficient. It should be noted that both vomiting (common in the first trimester), which hinders drug absorption, and increases in volemia (particularly in the second half of pregnancy), make it necessary to adjust the dosage according to the needs in each moment [57].

Plasma exchange plays an important role in the management of MG during pregnancy, fundamentally for the treatment and prevention of attacks and for avoiding the use of immunosuppressive drugs that could have teratogenic effects upon the fetus [58]. Plasmapheresis is the fastest option for controlling the effects upon the motor end plate, by removing the circulating autoantibodies [59] - though some authors associate it with the potential occurrence of preterm delivery [60].

The treatment of MG during pregnancy has included corticosteroids, mainly prednisone and azathioprine. The use of prednisone has been associated with an incidence of cleft palate of under 1%. Azathioprine should be avoided during pregnancy (grade of recommendation D), though no specific teratogenic effects profile has been associated with its use. Nevertheless, exposed fetuses have shown a certain tendency to develop anemia, thrombocytopenia, and transient leukopenia [61]. Other immunosuppressive agents such as methotrexate should be avoided. The introduction of monoclonal antibodies such as rituximab (targeted to B lymphocytes), belimumab (targeted to B cell activating factor), eculizumab (targeted to complement), or alefacept (targeted to T cell activation) opens new therapeutic options [62], though their safety and efficacy during pregnancy must be clarified.

When a patient receiving immunosuppressive therapy due to MG becomes pregnant, possible worsening of the condition must be considered when such therapy is discontinued. The risk/benefit ratio of maintaining treatment must be evaluated on an individualized basis.

The onset of delivery is not influenced by the disease, since the smooth muscle is not affected. Weakness and fatigue may develop during the second period of delivery, and can be treated with acetylcholine esterase inhibitors. Cesarean section should only be indicated for obstetric reasons, and general anesthesia is to be avoided. Epidural anesthesia is safe in these patients.

Twenty percent of the born infants will suffer a form of neonatal MG secondary to the transplacental transmission of antibodies. The severity of the condition is variable and unpredictable, though it tends to resolve between the first and fourth month of life. The transplacental transmission of antibodies can trigger congenital multiple arthrogryposis in the fetus due to the joint stiffness conditioned by the lack of mobility. This neonatal condition may even occur in relation to women with mild MG, and frequently recurs in subsequent pregnancies. Although few studies have been conducted to date, plasmapheresis during the first trimester may prevent its development [63].

Isoimmunization

When the mother and fetus present blood group incompatibility, maternal antibodies may form (isoimmunization), cross the placental barrier and bind to the fetal red blood cells, causing their destruction and producing what is known as hemolytic disease in the fetus or newborn infant.

There are many red cell surface antigens, though the great majority of those involved in this disease form part of the ABO system, and particularly the Rh system – specifically, antigen D.

The Rh system comprises 5 different antigens (C, c, D, E and e). Both antigens C and c and antigens E and e are alternate forms of the same antigen, in contrast to antigen D, which may or may not be present. This is what we refer to when a patient is described as being Rh D positive or Rh D negative.

Other antigen groups (Kell, Duffy, Kidd, MNS, Lutheran, P, etc.) also may be implicated in isoimmunization, but not all of them have the same clinical relevance.

As a cause of isoimmunization, the most frequent antibodies are anti-RhD, followed by anti-Rhc and anti-Kell antibodies. The rest of antigens are a very infrequent cause of isoimmunization.

Isoimmunization due to ABO system incompatibility is of scant clinical relevance, since in most cases there is no clinical expression, and when manifestations do occur they are usually of little importance (neonatal anemia and mild hyperbilirubinemia).

Frequency

Between 1-10% of all Rh negative mothers become sensitized after first pregnancy, 30% after second pregnancy, and 50% after third pregnancy. With the introduction of prophylaxis and improved means for the control and monitorization of pregnancy, it has become possible to greatly reduce the number of sensitized women, and therefore the incidence of fetal or neonatal hemolytic disease.

Specifically, following the introduction of prophylaxis, isoimmunization D decreased from 9.1-10.3 cases to only 1.3 cases per 1000 births.

Outcome and Clinical Manifestations

In situations characterized by an RhD negative mother with an Rh positive fetus (due to inheritance of the antigen from the father), a number of events may trigger maternal sensitization and thus isoimmunization, such as: delivery, labor, a threat of fetal loss, miscarriage, ectopic pregnancy, metrorrhagia in the third trimester (placental detachment, placenta previa, etc.), the use of invasive techniques (amniocentesis, chorial biopsy, etc.), abdominal trauma, or external cephalic version.

Sensitization may also occur in other processes external to pregnancy, such as: transfusions, handling objects contaminated with blood, organ transplantation, etc., since very little blood (< 0.1 ml) is needed to produce sensitization.

As in all antibody-mediated immune responses, isoimmunization is characterized by an initial production of IgM antibodies that are unable to cross the placental barrier. As a result, fetal or neonatal hemolytic disease is unlikely to develop in the same pregnancy in which sensitization has occurred.

However, in a second pregnancy, or in a woman previously sensitized via other means, the placental crossing of only a minimum amount of fetal blood can trigger a faster maternal immune response of greater magnitude, producing IgM but also IgG, which in turn can reach the fetal bloodstream and bind to the fetal erythrocytes. Once a certain amount of antigen has bound to an erythrocyte, the latter is destroyed through the complement pathway, with the production of hemolysis.

Hemolysis releases bilirubin, which the fetus excretes together with its degradation products in urine. Excessive bilirubin accumulation can give rise to nuclear jaundice, characterized by the formation of bilirubin deposits in the basal nuclei of the brain, with neurological symptoms.

Fetal anemia, which occurs when hemolysis exceeds the fetal hematopoietic capacity, induces the intervention of non-bone marrow hematopoiesis in the liver, with a reduction of the hepatic production of other proteins. As a consequence, the oncotic pressure within the fetal vascularization decreases. This drop in oncotic pressure, and the cardiac alterations associated with severe anemia (heart failure secondary to high output plus myocardial ischemia with dysfunction) result in an increase in fluid in the extravascular compartments: pericardial effusion, pleural effusion, ascites or subcutaneous edema. If at least two of these compartments are affected, fetal hydrops develops.

The normal tendency of isoimmunization is to worsen in subsequent pregnancies, due to immune system memory, and fetal anemia can develop at the same or earlier gestational age as in previously affected pregnancies.

Diagnosis and Treatment

The first prenatal evaluation of a pregnant woman should include determination of the ABO group and RhD group, along with an antierythrocyte antibodies screening test (Coombs' test) – the latter being repeated every trimester in Rh-negative patients.

If this screening test proves positive for anti-Lewis or anti-I antibodies, no expansion of the study is needed, since these antibodies are not related to fetal hemolytic disease.

However, if other antierythrocyte antibodies are identified, the study should be completed with antibody titration. The potency of the maternal antibody response can be assessed by antibody titration, though the latter does not inform us of the fetal status. Nevertheless, we can assume a significant risk of fetal hemolytic disease or hydrops beyond what is known as the critical titer (between 1/8 and 1/32).

The determination of bilirubin in amniotic fluid through amniocentesis can also be used, but this technique has been displaced by a less invasive procedure involving Doppler ultrasound measurement of the maximum (systolic) velocity of the middle cerebral artery (MCA-SV).

Table 2. MCA-SV values according to gestational age [64]

Gestational Age (weeks)	MCA-PSV (cm/s)	
	Median	**1,5 MoM**
14	19.3	28.9
15	20.2	30.3
16	21.1	31.7
17	22.1	33.2
18	23.2	34.8
19	24.3	36.5
20	25.5	38.2
21	26.7	40.0
22	27.9	41.9
23	29.3	43.9
24	30.7	46.0
25	32.1	48.2
26	33.6	50.4
27	35.2	52.8
28	36.9	55.4
29	38.7	58.0
30	40.5	60.7
31	42.4	63.6
32	44.4	66.6
33	46.5	69.8
34	48.7	73.1
35	51.1	76.6
36	53.5	80.2
37	56.0	84.0
38	58.7	88.9
39	61.5	92.2
40	64.4	96.6

As the hematocrit decreases, MCA-SV increases, and reference tables (Table 2) are used to identify the normal MCA-SV values according to gestational age [64].

Ultrasound can also be used to assess the presence or absence of fetal hydrops. In this context, the hematocrit value is usually below 15% in the presence of hydrops (Table 3).

If Doppler ultrasound indicates a risk of anemia (MCA-SV > 1.5 multiples of the median (MoM)), or the ultrasound study reveals the existence of fetal hydrops, cordocentesis must be performed, consisting of direct ultrasound measurement of the fetal hematocrit in umbilical vein blood. The fetal hematocrit is normally 36-44%, and in the presence of severe anemia this percentage drops to below 30%.

Management of Isoimmunization with Atypical Antigens

Antibodies such as anti-C, anti-K, anti-PP1Pk and anti-E, which potentially are able to cause severe fetal hemolytic disease, are dealt with in a way similar to anti-D isoimmunization, though the rest of antibodies do not require such detailed monitoring and study.

Table 3. Method for the measurement of middle cerebral artery systolic velocity (Gratacos E et al., 2007)

Method for the measurement of MCA-SV
• Fetus at rest and mother in apnea. • Axial section of the fetal skull at the level of the sphenoid bone. • Visualization of the circle of Willis using color Doppler. • It is necessary to expand the image so that the MCA closest to the transducer occupies over 50% of the screen. The MCA should be visualized over its entire length. • The cursor should be placed close to the origin of the MCA, and the ultrasound angle should be as close as possible to 0 degrees. Angle correction should not be used. • The waves (between 5-10) should be similar, with measurement of the highest peak systolic. • Fetal skull compression is to be avoided, as this may affect the Doppler spectrum. • MCA velocity is expressed in cm/s, and is converted to multiples of the median (MoM); it also can be expressed in standard deviations. • Repetition in triplicate is advised, using the mean for final calculation.

Gratacós E, Gómez R, Nicolaides K, Romero R, Cabrero L. Medicina Fetal. Editorial. Médica Panamericana; 2007.

The prevention of isoimmunization is based on the administration of anti-D gammaglobulin in Rh-negative mothers approximately in week 28 for prophylactic purposes, and following those abovementioned events that are able to induce sensitization: delivery or cesarean section of an Rh-positive fetus, miscarriage, ectopic pregnancy, metrorrhagia in the third trimester (placental detachment, placenta previa, etc.), the use of invasive techniques (amniocentesis, chorial biopsy, etc.), abdominal trauma, external cephalic version, or intrauterine fetal death [65].

An intramuscular dose of 300 μg of anti-D gammaglobulin should be administered in the first 72 hours of the sensitizing process. In those cases where fetal-maternal transfusion is > 30 ml, the dose should be adjusted according to the degree of fetal-maternal bleeding estimated by the Kleihauer test, HbF determination or flow cytometry. A 20 μg dose of anti-D gammaglobulin per ml of fetal-maternal bleeding is indicated.

Treatment mainly consists of correcting the fetal anemia through intrauterine fetal transfusions directly into the umbilical vein, following cordocentesis to determine the true fetal hematocrit value. It is generally agreed that transfusion should be performed when anemia is moderate or severe (-4 standard deviations (SD)), or when the hematocrit is < 30%.

The volume of erythrocytes to be transfused is calculated from the estimated fetal weight, gestational age, hematocrit of the blood unit, the actual fetal hematocrit and the desired hematocrit. After 2-3 transfusions, most circulating erythrocytes in the fetus are Rh-negative.

Use of Plasmapheresis in Isoimmunization

Since intrauterine transfusion (first-line treatment) requires a certain gestational age in order to minimize the risks of the procedure, the use of apheretic techniques, together with the administration of intravenous immunoglobulins, has been postulated as a treatment option in early gestational periods, based on the fact that they result in antibody clearance with a drop in titers, and therefore in the number of destroyed erythrocytes [66].

According to the 2013 clinical guide of the American Society for Apheresis (ASFA) [5], plasmapheresis in the treatment of isoimmunization corresponds to category III (Table 4), which includes those conditions for which the role of apheresis has not been established. According to the ASFA, apheresis has grade of recommendation 2C (Table 5), and its use is to be accepted in cases in which the gestational age does not yet allow safe intrauterine transfusion.

According to some studies [67, 68] involving cases at a high risk of fetal complications due to a history of fetal losses, severe isoimmunization or high antibody titers, plasmapheresis was able to lower the antibody titers, though intrauterine transfusion finally proved necessary. They therefore concluded that plasmapheresis and intravenous immunoglobulin administration are adequate for the management of severe isoimmunization.

However, a case has also been reported [69] involving elevated antibodies in which plasmapheresis and intravenous immunoglobulin were used throughout pregnancy, affording adequate control of the disease without the need for intrauterine fetal transfusion. In another similar case [70], plasmapheresis and intravenous immunoglobulin made it possible to reach an advanced gestational age, though signs of severe anemia (as evidenced by Doppler MCA-SV and ultrasonographic signs of hydrops) led to the decision to discontinue pregnancy.

Regarding isoimmunization involving atypical antigens [71], plasmapheresis in a case of anti-K antibodies and in a case of anti-PP-1Pk positivity resulted in a satisfactory course, with reduced antibody titers and no apparent fetal complications.

Table 4. Categories of the American Society for Apheresis (ASFA) [66]

Category	Description
I	Disorders for which apheresis is accepted as first-line therapy, either as a primary standalone treatment or in conjunction with other modes of treatment. Example: plasma exchange in Guillain-Barre syndrome as 1st-line standalone therapy; plasma exchange in myasthenia gravis as 1st-line in conjunction with immunosuppression and cholinesterase inhibition
II	Disorders for which apheresis is accepted as secondline therapy, either as a standalone treatment or in conjunction with other modes of treatment. Example: plasma exchange as standalone secondary treatment for acute disseminated encephalomyelitis after high-dose IV corticosteroid failure; extracorporeal photopheresis added to corticosteroids for unresponsive chronic graft-versus-host disease
III	Optimum role of apheresis therapy is not established. Decision making should be individualized. Example: extracorporeal photopheresis for nephrogenic systemic fibrosis; plasma exchange in patients with sepsis and multi-organ failure
IV	Disorders in which published evidence demonstrates or suggests apheresis to be ineffective or harmful. IRB approval is desirable if apheresis treatment is undertaken in these circumstances. Example: plasma exchange for active rheumatoid arthritis

Table 5. Grading Recommendations adapted from Guyatt et al.

Recommendation	Description	Methodological quality of supporting evidence	Implications
Grade 1A	Strong recommendation, high-quality evidence	RCTs without important limitations or overwhelming evidence from observational studies	Strong recommendation, can apply to most patients in most circumstances without reservation
Grade 1B	Strong recommendation, Moderate quality evidence	RCTs with important limitations or exceptionally strong evidence from observational studies	Strong recommendation, can apply to most patients in most circumstances without reservation
Grade 1C	Strong recommendation, low quality evidence	Observational studies or case series	Strong recommendation but may change when higher quality evidence becomes available
Grade 2A	Weak recommendation, high quality evidence	RCTs without important limitations or overwhelming evidence from observational studies	Weak recommendation, best action may differ depending on circumstances or patients'or societal values
Grade 2B	Weak recommendation, moderate-quality evidence	RCTs with important limitations or exceptionally strong evidence from observational studies	Weak recommendation, best action may differ depending on circumstances or patients' or societal values
Grade 2C	Weak recommendation, low-quality or very low-quality evidence	Observational studies or case series	Very weak recommendations; other alternatives may be equally reasonable

Guyatt, Gordon H., et al. "Rating quality of evidence and strength of recommendations: GRADE: an emerging consensus on rating quality of evidence and strength of recommendations." BMJ: British Medical Journal 336.7650 (2008): 924.

Although further studies are needed, it can be concluded that the prescription of plasmapheresis for the management of isoimmunization should center on early gestational ages in which it is not yet possible to perform intrauterine transfusions [66], and on cases characterized by a high risk of fetal complications [67, 68].

Antiphospholipid Syndrome

Antiphospholipid syndrome (APS) is a systemic autoimmune disease characterized by acquired hypercoagulability, with the occurrence of thromboembolic events and/or obstetric complications in the presence of persistent intermediate or high titers of antiphospholipid antibodies such as anticardiolipin IgG or IgM, anti-β2-glycoprotein IgG or IgM, or lupus anticoagulant.

The condition is classified as either primary APS (50% of all cases), in the absence of clinical or biological manifestations of any other disease, or secondary APS, associated mainly to systemic lupus erythematosus (SLE)(20-35% of all patients with SLE will develop secondary APS), or to other autoimmune disorders [72, 73].

Catastrophic antiphospholipid syndrome (CAPS) is an infrequent acute variant of the disorder (representing < 1% of all cases of APS), characterized by massive microangiopathy and multiorgan failure. It was first described by Asherson [74] in 1992.

Certain predisposing factors capable of triggering such an acute condition have been reported in 50% [75] of the cases: infections (22%), surgery (10%), drugs such as oral contraceptives (7%), obstetric complications (7%), neoplasms (5%) and SLE (3%). However, it is not fully clear why a small percentage of patients with APS will develop CAPS [76]. The mortality rate is close to 30% in the absence of adequate treatment, and is fundamentally attributable to acute myocardial infarction [75].

Antiphospholipid syndrome affects mainly young women (between 20-40 years of age) with a 3.5:1 female: male ratio in the case of primary APS and a 7:1 ratio in the case of APS secondary to SLE [73].

Some authors suggest that the syndrome is the most common acquired hypercoagulability state and affects over 2% of the population.

However, not all patients with circulating antibodies develop the clinical features of the syndrome, since antiphospholipid antibodies are present in 5% of the healthy population [77].

Clinical Manifestations

Antiphospholipid syndrome is characterized by systemic thromboembolic phenomena, obstetric complications, and possible thrombocytopenia.

Thrombosis may be of either arterial or venous origin, though venous thrombosis is more common and is typically located in the extremities with or without associated pulmonary (PTE), renal, hepatic and retinal thromboembolism. In turn, arterial thrombosis most often exhibits a coronary, renal, and mesenteric distribution [78].

Pregnant patients suffer thrombosis of the placental vascularization. In this context, several studies have shown antiphospholipid antibodies to bind to trophoblastic cells, triggering a local inflammatory response through activation of the coagulation cascade and complement system [6]. The antibodies thus appear to be the direct cause of trophoblastic dysfunction and complement activation at the fetal-maternal interface, resulting in a deficient exchange of components between the maternal and fetal blood, with consequent obstetric complications related to APS: miscarriage, preeclampsia, restricted intrauterine growth, and even intrauterine fetal death [79].

Table 6. Revised classification criteria for definite APS [75]

Clinical criteria (1 or more of the following)	Laboratory criteria (1 or more of the following present on 2 or more occasions at least 12 weeks apart using recommended procedures)
Vascular thrombosis: 1 or more objectively confirmed episodes of arterial, venous **or** small vessel thrombosis occurring in any tissue or organ **Pregnancy morbidity**: 1 or more unexplained deaths of a morphologically normal fetus at or beyond the 10th week of gestation; **or** 1 or more premature births of a morphologically normal neonate before the 34th week of gestation because of eclampsia, preeclampsia, or placental insufficiency; **or** 3 or more unexplained consecutive spontaneous abortions before the 10th week of gestation	**LA** detected according to the guidelines of the ISTH **ACL antibody** of IgG and/or IgM isotype, present in medium **or** high titer (40 IgG or IgM phospholipid units or >99th percentile) measured by a standardized ELISA Anti–β2GPI antibody of IgG and/or IgM isotype present in titer > 99th percentile measured by a standardized ELISA

Diagnosis

Antiphospholipid syndrome (APS) should be suspected in women of childbearing potential who suffer thromboembolic events and/or recurrent miscarriage or other obstetric complications in the apparent absence of risk factors.

A number of clinical and laboratory criteria are used to diagnose APS, and were last revised in Sydney in 2006 [80]. The presence of a clinical criterion together with a laboratory criterion is required in order to establish a diagnosis of APS (Table 6).

Other antibodies are very common but are not specific of APS, and so are not included among the diagnostic criteria:

- Anticardiolipin IgA
- Anti-β2-glycoprotein IgA
- Antiphosphatidylserine
- Antiphosphatidyl ethanolamine
- Specific antibodies targeted to prothrombin
- Phosphatidylserine-prothrombin complex

Diagnostic Criteria of Catastrophic Antiphospholipid Syndrome (CAPS) [5]

1) Evidence of alterations affecting three or more organs, systems or tissues
2) Development of manifestations either simultaneously or in under one week
3) Histological confirmation of small vessel thrombosis in at least one organ or tissue
4) Laboratory test confirmation of the presence of antiphospholipid antibodies

All four criteria must be met in order to establish a firm diagnosis of CAPS, since less than four is only indicative of probable CAPS.

Peculiarities of APS in Pregnancy

The relationship between APS and pregnancy is so intimate that obstetric complications form part of the clinical diagnostic criteria of the syndrome. A more in-depth description therefore will be offered below regarding the particularities of both the clinical manifestations and the diagnosis and treatment of APS during pregnancy.

The most common obstetric complications in patients with APS are recurrent miscarriage, restricted intrauterine growth, preeclampsia, HELLP syndrome, abruptio placentae and fetal death [81, 82]. Such complications in turn are more common in patients with triple antiphospholipid antibody positivity [73].

- Miscarriage: Recurrent miscarriage in APS is of such importance that it constitutes one of the clinical criteria for establishing the diagnosis, and is the most frequent obstetric complication of the syndrome. Van den Boogaard et al. [81] considered APS to be responsible for 18% of all recurrent miscarriages, after excluding other possible causes.
- Intrauterine growth restriction (IUGR): The big problem in knowing the exact relationship between IUGR and APS is that the criteria used in defining IUGR have changed a lot in recent years, and no consensus has been established. One of the most widely accepted criteria in recent years is that IUGR can be assumed in situations of percentile fetal growth < 3 or between 3-10, but accompanied by changes in brain-umbilical or uterine artery flow values. What does seem clear is the cause of IUGR, because we know that the APS is implicated in trophoblastic invasion problems, which in the event of ongoing pregnancy could cause placental insufficiency with consequent fetal growth restriction. Thus, different prevalence values are obtained, depending on the series analyzed and on the criteria used to define IUGR. Nevertheless, the Euro-Phospholipid Project reports a 26.3% incidence of IUGR in pregnant women with APS [83].
- Preeclampsia: This condition is defined by the presence of arterial hypertension beyond week 20 of pregnancy, accompanied by proteinuria. A distinction can be made among preeclampsia, severe preeclampsia, and the most fatal form of the disorder, known as eclampsia, which is characterized by the presence of seizures. In reference to the above described physiopathological mechanism, it

seems that the same trophoblastic invasion problems may also cause preeclampsia.

Based on the current literature, it is difficult to establish the relationship between preeclampsia and APS, since most available studies make no distinction among the different degrees of severity within preeclampsia. Nevertheless, the Euro-Phospholipid Project reports a 9.5% incidence of preeclampsia in pregnant women with APS [82].

- HELLP syndrome:
  - Hemolysis: damaged red blood cells, with a consequent increase in bilirubin and yellow coloring of the skin (jaundice) in the case of very high bilirubin concentrations.
  - Lowered platelet counts: between 150,000-100,000 (HELLP class III), between 100,000-50,000 (HELLP class II), or under 50,000 (HELLP class I).
  - In addition, HELLP syndrome is characterized by liver alterations, with elevated liver enzymes and transaminases.

HELLP syndrome can manifest isolatedly or, more commonly, as a complication of preeclampsia. Patients with established preeclampsia and HELLP syndrome are at an increased risk of developing CAPS, as demonstrated by Hanouna et al. [84] in a retrospective study in which 12 out of 13 cases of CAPS during pregnancy were seen to have been preceded by preeclampsia and HELLP syndrome. The clinical criteria are described in Table 3 [85, 86, 87].

Treatment

Before describing the treatment of APS, it must be underscored that the first step towards good control of the disease is to ensure thorough preconception counseling with a view to programming pregnancy from a multidisciplinary perspective, with the participation of different specialists involved in the management of such patients. Such an approach is not always possible, however, and in some cases APS is diagnosed as a result of some adverse effect occurring during pregnancy.

Following the above consideration, a first question is raised: Should we treat those patients with positive antiphospholipid antibodies but no history of thrombosis or adverse obstetric events?

According to the most recent literature, there is no recommendation to treat these patients [88], since the risk of thrombosis is similar to that observed among pregnant women without antiphospholipid antibodies [89, 90]. This criterion is documented in the guidelines for the treatment of APS of the Brazilian Society of Rheumatology [88].

First Line Treatment

First line treatment in pregnant women already diagnosed with APS comprises dual therapy based on low-dose aspirin, starting treatment when the patient seeks to become pregnant (hence the importance of preconception counseling in these patients), and on low-molecular weight heparin (LMWH) – starting administration when a positive pregnancy test is obtained [88].

If no first line treatment for APS is provided, a favorable course of pregnancy is observed in only about 20% of the cases. In contrast, with adequate first line treatment, pregnancy to term can be observed in up to 70% of the cases [91].

Second Line Treatment

Second line treatment is used to complement first line therapy with a view to securing benefits in certain cases where the treatment of choice alone is not enough.

The main problem is that the experience gained with second line treatment, as established from clinical trials and publications, is much more limited.

Second line treatment comprises the following therapies [91, 92]:

- Corticosteroids
- Hydroxychloroquine
- Intravenous immunoglobulins
- Plasmapheresis
- B-cell targeted therapies: rituximab
- Anti-TNF-α therapies: infliximab, etanercept and adalimumab

Treatment of Catastrophic Antiphospholipid Syndrome (CAPS)

Catastrophic antiphospholipid syndrome has a high mortality rate (close to 30%) in the absence of optimum treatment. It is therefore essential to not delay the management of such cases.

- A first requirement is to treat the triggering factors whenever possible (infections, drugs, etc.).
- As a second step, treatment should include high-dose anticoagulants, corticosteroids, and plasmapheresis and/or intravenous immunoglobulins [93].

However, the prescription of cyclophosphamide, which in some cases has also been included in the therapeutic protocol, is controversial, since it has not been able to demonstrate benefits [94].

Use of Plasmapheresis

As has been seen above, there is greater consensus on the indication of apheresis during pregnancy in catastrophic antiphospholipid syndrome (CAPS) than in antiphospholipid syndrome itself.

Although the precise mechanism of action has not been established, it seems that plasmapheresis is of help in the management of CAPS because it is able to eliminate antiphospholipid antibodies, cytokines, TNF and complement. On the other hand, the replacement plasma used contains natural anticoagulants such as antithrombin and proteins C and S [93].

According to the 2010 clinical guide of the American Society for Apheresis (ASFA) and its subsequent update in 2013 [93], plasmapheresis in the treatment of CAPS corresponds to category II (Table 4), which includes those conditions where apheresis is accepted as second line treatment. However, in the 2007 edition of the guide, plasmapheresis was assigned to category III, which includes those conditions for which the role of apheresis has not been established. Considering the evolution of the category in recent years, it can be concluded that the indication of plasmapheresis in the management of CAPS is increasingly accepted and supported by scientific evidence.

The largest study published to date [94] on the indication of plasmapheresis in CAPS, involving 250 cases, concluded that the combination of anticoagulants, corticosteroids and plasmapheresis should be regarded as first line treatment, since it shows a clear increase in survival rate among patients with CAPS.

Regarding antiphospholipid syndrome, some studies [95] have found plasmapheresis to be effective in reducing the antibody titers in pregnant women with CAPS, but have been unable to confirm an impact upon the clinical manifestations. In contrast, another publication [96] has reported that plasmapheresis reduces the antibody titers, and this in turn leads to an improved perinatal outcome.

Other studies [97] of the indication of plasmapheresis in high risk APS subgroups (patients with a history of thromboembolic events, triple positive antibodies, etc.) have concluded that plasmapheresis combined with other therapies such as intravenous immunoglobulins is acceptable as second line treatment for the management of these patients.

The literature on the subject and the recommendations of the ASFA [93] indicate that plasmapheresis is openly accepted for the management of CAPS and also for APS in those clinical situations in which first line treatment proves insufficient.

Systemic Lupus Erythematosus

Systemic lupus erythematosus (SLE) is a chronic, multisystemic autoimmune disease of unknown origin characterized by the appearance of inflammatory phenomena that can affect multiple body systems, with a tendency towards alternating periods of remission and relapse. As a result, the course and prognosis of the disease vary greatly depending on the form of presentation [98].

Systemic lupus erythematosus shows a strong predominance among females, particularly during the reproductive stage of life. It is therefore important to study the interaction between SLE and pregnancy. The disease affects one out of every 1000 women of childbearing potential, between the second and fourth decade of life. In turn, SLE shows a greater incidence and severity in Negro and Asian women [99].

Pregnancy in women with SLE can be complicated by both the activity of the disease itself, and by the effect of the physiological changes of pregnancy upon the natural course of SLE. Most recent studies describe an increase in SLE activity during pregnancy, perhaps exacerbated by the hormonal changes [100]. Similarly, increased activity of the disease has a negative impact upon pregnancy - the risk of problems being greater in patients who have had SLE activity in the 6 months before pregnancy, as well as in the presence of kidney disease [101].

Clinical Manifestations during Pregnancy

One of the aspects that proves most difficult to assess is the activity of the disease during pregnancy, since it is not easy to establish a differential diagnosis among the physiological changes, preeclampsia, and HELLP syndrome (Tables 7 and 8). There are no clear data on the frequency of acute SLE flare-ups during pregnancy, since some studies report an increased incidence, while others describe a frequency of flare-ups similar to that observed in non-pregnant women. Likewise, the time of greatest flare-up frequency during pregnancy has not been established.

Table 7. Clinical criteria for diagnosis [85, 87]

Severe Preeclampsia ACOG criteria. (any of these findings)	– Systolic blood pressure of 160 mm Hg or higher, or diastolic blood pressure of 110 mm Hg or higher on two occasions at least 4 hours apart while the patient is on bed rest – Cerebral or visual disturbances – Pulmonary edema – Trombocytopenia (platelets count less than 100×10^9/L – Impaired liver function as indicated by abnormally elevated blood concentrations of liver enzymes (to twice normal concentration), severe persistent right upper quadrant or epigastric pain unresponsive to medication and not accounted for by alternative diagnoses, or both – Progressive renal insuffiency (serum creatinine concentration greater than 1.1 mg/dl or a doubling of the serum creatinine concentration in the absence of other renal disease
HELLP Mississippi criteria	– Thrombocytopenia (usually $<100 \times 10^9$/L) with a documented prenatally normal platelet count – Hepatic dysfunction: AST> 48 IU/L, ALT > 24 IU/L or LDH>164 IU/L – Evidence of intravascular hemolysis, to include a decreasing hematocrit concurrent with worsening thrombocytopenia, an increase in LDH, and/or evidence of bleeding involving intravenous sites or hematuria – No evidence of another disorder primarily causative of clinical and laboratory findings

Table 8. Differential diagnosis of lupus nephritis, preeclampsia, and HELLP syndrome [121]

	Physiological changes	Lupus nephritis	Preeclampsia	HELLP syndrome
Appearance	Any time	Any time	Gestational age > 20w	Gestational age > 34w
Anemia	Non-hemolytic	Hemolytic	Usually absent	Microangiopathic
Thrombocytopenia	8% counts < 10^5	Normal or decreased	Normal or decreased	Counts < 10^5
Creatinine	Decreased	Normal or increased	Normal or increased	Normal
Proteinuria	Normal	Normal or increased	> 300 mg/24 h	Normal or increased
Liver function	Normal	Normal	Normal or increased	Increased
Blood pressure	Normal	Normal or increased	Increased	Normal or increased
Complement	Increased	Normal or decreased	Normal	Normal
Anti-dsDNA antibodies	Negative	Increased	Negative	Negative

One of the aspects that conditions the risk of relapse during pregnancy is the symptoms-free period before conception. A relapse-free period of 6-12 months before pregnancy is recommended, since poor control of the disease, as well as sudden treatment discontinuation, are associated with adverse obstetric and maternal outcomes. It must be taken into account that the disease may first manifest with pregnancy in patients presenting subclinical SLE [102].

Active disease may be present in approximately 40-50% of all pregnant women with SLE - the most common manifestations being lupus nephritis, skin disease, osteoarthritis and hematological disorders (especially thrombocytopenia). In this context, over 75% of all patients with lupus symptoms will suffer kidney disease in the future. [103]

It is not easy to distinguish the acute symptoms of SLE from the physiological changes of pregnancy, since joint pain, fatigue, melasma, postpartum hair loss, breathing difficulties, edema and headache can often occur during normal pregnancy [104]. Relative anemia may be normal in pregnancy, though not so hemolytic anemia, which is typical of active SLE. Another element that can help differentiate physiological changes from active SLE is the serum complement values, as these tend to increase in normal pregnancy but either decrease or remain constant in active SLE. Likewise, active SLE is characterized by elevated anti-dsDNA antibody titers [105].

Another important aspect that must be taken into account is the differential diagnosis between lupus nephritis and preeclampsia and HELLP syndrome. In this context, lupus nephritis is often associated with hemolytic anemia, increased creatinine levels and proteinuria, while the blood pressure values and liver function parameters tend to remain stable. In contrast, preeclampsia is usually characterized by increased pressure values, proteinuria and altered liver function, while HELLP syndrome is typically associated with microangiopathic hemolytic anemia, thrombocytopenia, and altered liver function [106]. Differentiation is not easy, particularly in patients with subclinical SLE who suffer a disease flare-up, or in patients with manifestations of preeclampsia added to lupus disease. In some cases a renal biopsy is required to establish the differential diagnosis, though this technique implies an increased risk of bleeding.

Regarding the laboratory test findings related to SLE activity, the complement levels (C3 and C4) may decrease in situations of increased SLE activity, since these proteins are consumed in the inflammatory process. In pregnancy, however, the complement levels can increase 10-50% secondary to the increase in liver protein synthesis. Thus, the usefulness of complement measurement in pregnancy is not clear. Isolated lowering of the blood complement levels is not particularly predictive of SLE activity.

Antibodies targeted to double-strand DNA (dsDNA) are highly sensitive in diagnosing SLE, and may help identify increased lupus activity, particularly in the context of kidney disease. An increase in dsDNA levels during pregnancy may reflect increased disease activity [107]. The erythrocyte sedimentation rate (ESR) is unreliable in pregnancy, however, since it increases significantly in normal pregnancy. In contrast, C-reactive protein (CRP) may be more useful. C-reactive protein does not increase in all pregnancies, and may be more representative of the degree of general inflammation. In normal pregnancies, increased CRP in the second trimester has been associated with premature delivery. In non-pregnant patients with SLE, the CRP concentrations may increase during a lupus flare-up. The use of CRP has not yet been systematically tested in pregnant patients with SLE.

Lupus Nephritis

Renal involvement in SLE is defined as lupus nephritis, and is observed in 50% of all patients. Nevertheless, virtually all patients would show glomerular lesions if immunofluorescence techniques were used. The histological forms range from several types of glomerulonephritis to renal sclerosis. Renal problems are the manifestations that most condition the prognosis of the disease.

A number of studies have been made to determine whether pregnancy worsens renal function in patients with SLE. It is generally accepted that kidney disease flare-ups can occur during pregnancy, though these are generally mild or moderate. As has been commented above, the percentage risk of lupus nephritis during pregnancy ranges from 4-30%, depending on the series. Women with a history of lupus nephritis have a 20-30% risk of relapse during pregnancy. Among the women who suffer renal functional impairment due to lupus nephritis during pregnancy, an estimated 25% will have permanent renal damage despite aggressive treatment - though very few patients require dialysis for life. Such problems are more common in women with active disease at the time of conception.

It is important to assess renal activity during pregnancy. Urinary protein excretion is normally increased during pregnancy as a result of increased glomerular filtration, and this limits its usefulness in assessing renal function. For the same reason, creatinine concentration also decreases, and the usefulness of this parameter is therefore also limited. In this context, two aspects are important in detecting renal failure:

Serum creatinine should remain stable during pregnancy, since creatinine elevation could be a sign of renal failure.

Doubling of the baseline proteinuria levels in pregnant women with lupus who already have prior renal damage is indicative of renal failure.

Patients with lupus nephritis have an increased risk of complications during pregnancy. Consequently, pregnancy should be avoided until there has been renal disease remission for at least 6 months. Ideally, pregnancy should be postponed until after 12-18 months of remission [107, 108].

Adverse Effects upon Pregnancy

- *Pregnancy loss:* In general, approximately 20% of all pregnancies in women with SLE end in miscarriage (spontaneous abortion) or fetal death [108]. The risk of miscarriage is not much higher than in the general population, though, the risk of late fetal loss is greater. The two most important risk factors for pregnancy loss are increased SLE activity (particularly renal disease) and antiphospholipid syndrome (APS). In general, the live newborn rate is lower than in the general population.

- *Premature delivery:* The risk of premature delivery (i.e., delivery before week 37 of pregnancy) is estimated to be 33% in patients with SLE. Premature membrane rupture is an important cause of premature delivery among patients with SLE [109, 110]. Most premature births are spontaneous, though a significant proportion are induced in the best interest of the mother or fetus, due to severe disease flare-up. The risk factors for premature delivery include SLE disease activity before and during pregnancy, prednisone dose escalation, thyroid disease, and arterial hypertension. One of the hypotheses regarding the pathogenesis of premature delivery in patients with SLE is the inflammatory stress applied to the uterus and placenta, causing an increase in premature delivery and membrane rupture.
- *Low birth weight:* Patients with SLE present an increased incidence (5-35%) of infants with low birth weight, probably in relation to placental failure [110]. No clear risk factors have been identified, though low birth weight might be related to placental insufficiency secondary to the increased incidence of thrombosis in pregnancies among women with SLE.

Similarly, maternal complications are more frequent during pregnancy, including increased mortality and a higher risk of sepsis and pneumonia, postpartum bleeding, anemia, thrombocytopenia and venous thromboembolism, as well as hypertensive states, diabetes, renal failure and thrombophilia [111].

Neonatal Lupus

Neonatal lupus (NL) is a diverse condition that can be observed in neonates born from a mother with SLE. Physiopathologically, NL is due to the transplacental transmission of IgG autoantibodies between weeks 12-16 of pregnancy, with action upon the fetal tissues. It has been shown that 98% of all cases of NL exhibit anti-Ro antibody positivity, while only 1-2% of all pregnant women with anti-Ro antibodies give birth to an infant with NL [112]. The disease can manifest with involvement of a single organ, or as a general disorder [112].

Heart Disease

Heart disease in NL can manifest as heart block, cardiomyopathy, or other arrhythmias or repolarization disorders. The most frequent cardiac manifestation is congenital heart block.

Congenital atrioventricular (AV) block usually develops between weeks 18-24 of pregnancy, and more rarely in later stages or during postpartum. It may present in all grades (I, II or II), and the diagnosis is usually established from fetal bradycardia in the context of complete block. The condition is not intrinsically associated to congenital cardiac abnormalities, since the fetal heart is morphologically formed by gestational week 12, and transplacental transmission occurs in later stages [113, 114]. In the absence of congenital cardiomyopathy, atrioventricular block is generally well tolerated by the fetus. Intrauterine death is usually associated with untreatable heart failure of sudden onset [114].

The *de novo* incidence rate is 1.3-2%, while recurrence in subsequent pregnancies is observed in 12-18% of the cases. The diagnosis is based on fetal echocardiography, with electrocardiographic confirmation after birth [113, 114]. An early diagnosis is important in order to distinguish between complete and incomplete block, since the latter may be a candidate for intrauterine treatment. Fetal echocardiography every two weeks between weeks 16-25 of pregnancy is advisable in high risk pregnancies.

With regard to prenatal treatment, fluorinated corticosteroids offer benefit in incomplete block, but are not recommended on a prophylactic basis, due to the possible maternal-fetal deleterious effects. Other proposed therapies include intravenous immunoglobulins, in order to reduce transplacental transmission and thus also recurrence, as well as plasmapheresis (both therapies currently being under study) [114]. After birth, treatment comprises pacemaker implantation or surgery, depending on patient tolerance and age.

Myocardiopathy manifests in a lesser percentage of cases, and may be independent of atrioventricular block. It can be either localized or diffuse. Myocardiopathy has a poor neonatal outcome, with a high mortality rate in the absence of treatment [113]. The condition can independently manifest as pericarditis – the diagnosis being established from the finding of pericardial effusion with no other signs of fetal hydrops.

Arrhythmias in the context of neonatal lupus can be transient or persistent, and include sick sinus disease, flutter, or prolongation of the QT-interval [114].

Skin manifestations in turn are observed in 15-25% of all cases of neonatal lupus. Such manifestations occasionally can be confused with other forms of neonatal rash, particularly in mothers who are not known to have SLE. A full 95% of the mothers are anti-Ro positive, although association of the latter with anti-La antibodies is usually greater than in cardiac lupus. Affected infants present photosensitive rash, though in some cases the lesions are located on unexposed areas. The skin manifestations usually develop after 4-6 weeks of life and persist for about 15 weeks, after which antibody clearance occurs [1115, 116]. The condition usually disappears without treatment.

Liver involvement is observed in 10-25% of all cases of NL. The liver alterations comprise severe liver failure, conjugated hyperbilirubinemia with or without transaminase elevation in the first weeks of life, or mild transaminase elevation at 2-3 months of age [115].

As regards hematological disorders, any of the blood cell lines can be affected, though thrombocytopenia is the most common finding. It shows an early onset, tends to resolve within 2-4 weeks, and has no clinical consequences. In some cases neutropenia can be observed, characterized by a later onset and without associated secondary infections. Hemolytic anemia, pancytopenia or aplastic anemia are observed in very rare instances [113].

Treatment

The management of acute flare-ups can be individualized according to severity and the type of organ affected. In general, immunosuppression with non-fluorinated glucocorticoids, azathioprine or cyclosporin poses only minimum risks.

All patients should maintain treatment with hydroxychloroquine, since fetal exposure during the first trimester of pregnancy has resulted in no increase in the incidence of malformations, while withdrawal of the drug duplicates the relapse rate. Hydroxychloroquine use is therefore justified. The most serious symptoms that have been controlled with hydroxychloroquine are osteoarthritis and constitutional symptoms, while other more severe manifestations such as thrombocytopenia and proteinuria are refractory to the drug [117, 118, 119].

In general, intraarticular corticosteroid injection may offer benefit in the event of active osteoarthritis affecting a limited number of joints.

Nonsteroidal antiinflammatory drugs (NSAIDs) in turn may be used during the first half of pregnancy, provided they are not associated with teratogenic effects. However, both selective and non-selective NSAIDs may alter fetal circulation though the inhibition of prostaglandin synthesis, leading to decreased fetal renal filtration, with the resulting dose-dependent oligoamnios. This phenomenon has been reported with indomethacin, ketoprofen, ibuprofen, and some COX-2 inhibitors. Severe neonatal renal failure may occur in the event of fetal exposure in the 72 hours leading to delivery. Likewise, early ductus closure has been reported, regardless of the administered dose, and mainly when the medication is administered after week 31, with a tendency to resolve within 24 hours after drug discontinuation. The administration of these drugs therefore should be limited to the first half of pregnancy, taking care to avoid prescription in the 8 weeks before delivery. Likewise, strict ultrasound control is required when these substances are administered on a chronic basis, in order to detect possible side effects [120]. COX-2 inhibitors are not recommended, since there are not enough data to confirm their safety during pregnancy.

Non-fluorinated glucocorticoids are commonly used to treat SLE. Their use during the first three months of pregnancy has been associated with palatal defects, while administration during the second and third trimesters has been related to hypertension and diabetes in the mother, and to low birth weight in the infant [121]. During the first trimester, prednisone should be kept below 15 mg/day, to ensure only 5-10% of free prednisone present in maternal plasma. After formation of the placenta, corticosteroids are partially inactivated by placental 11-β-hydroxylase, affording relative fetal protection. Towards the end of pregnancy, doses over 20 mg/day may increase the incidence of premature delivery.

No congenital malformations have been associated with the use of azathioprine. Intrauterine exposure to this drug can sometimes cause mild bone marrow suppression, reflected by leukopenia and thrombocytopenia at birth. In order to avoid the suppression of hematopoiesis, the dose should be maintained between 1.5-2 mg/kg/day. Azathioprine has also been related to an increase in prematurity and low birth weight [112]. Nevertheless, its use is justified in the case of moderate to severe flare-ups.

Exposure to cyclosporine has been associated with a 3% incidence of congenital malformations, though with no defined pattern. Furthermore, the incidence is no greater than that found in the general population. Cyclosporine has not been associated to altered liver or kidney function. The drug has been associated to premature delivery (40-46% of the cases) and low birth weight (44-65%).

As regards the use of cyclophosphamide, its effect upon human pregnancy may be unpredictable. The defects related to exposure in the first trimester comprise facial, musculoskeletal and visceral malformations, alterations in growth and development, and miscarriage following administration during the first trimester. Administration in the second half of pregnancy may cause pancytopenia in the newborn infant. It is therefore necessary to postpone pregnancy until three months after the suspension of cyclophosphamide [123].

The administration of intravenous immunoglobulins is indicated for the treatment of thrombocytopenia in the pregnant patient. No fetal adverse effects have been demonstrated [124].

Methotrexate and leflunomide are totally contraindicated, while insufficient data are available referred to the use of rituximab and other biological agents [125].

As a general rule, we can use the following treatment protocol [114]:

- Mild flare-ups (joint pain, osteoarthritis, serositis, skin rash): Oral corticosteroids at medium-low doses (< 20 mg/day) or NSAIDs used intermittently and at lower doses, during the last part of the first trimester and during the second trimester of pregnancy.
- Moderate to severe flare-ups: High-dose oral corticosteroids or intravenous corticosteroid pulses (0.5 mg/kg/day), azathioprine, cyclosporine, tacrolimus or intravenous immunoglobulins. It should be noted that the safety profile of intravenous corticosteroid pulses differs from that of oral administration, and acute fetal vasospasm, sudden hypertension and placental ischemia may result.
- Cyclophosphamide may be considered in the second and third trimesters in more severe cases, though fetal loss may occur.

Use of Plasmapheresis

In relation to new approaches in the management of SLE, different studies have shown plasmapheresis to improve the clinical manifestations of the disease [126, 127]. In effect, plasmapheresis is useful in situations of important thrombocytopenia, diffuse alveolar hemorrhage [128], lupus nephritis [129] or acute skin conditions [130], among other indications.

A recent study conducted by Stojan et al. [131] on the prevention, diagnosis and management of SLE flare-ups during pregnancy and in the puerperal period has examined the use of plasmapheresis as a treatment option in different situations. In the event of acute liver steatosis during pregnancy, our first concern is to end pregnancy as soon as the patient has been stabilized, generally through the administration of fresh frozen plasma (FFP) and other derivatives to treat blood imbalances and/or severe coagulopathy, and aggressive correction of hypoglycemia and electrolyte alterations. Thrombotic thrombocytopenic purpura (TTP) is treated with plasma exchange or plasmapheresis [132].

According to the American Society for Apheresis (ASFA), plasmapheresis in the treatment of SLE corresponds to category III, with grade of recommendation 2B. Both the category and the grade of recommendation vary according to the clinical presentation of the disease (Tables 9 and 10).

The frequency of therapeutic plasma exchange (PEX) depends on the clinical manifestations of the disease.

A number of studies, such as those mentioned above, report good results with plasma exchange for the treatment of SLE. Some authors combine plasmapheresis with drugs such as cyclosporine, prednisone or cyclophosphamide.

Regarding the duration, interval between sessions, and the number of required plasmapheresis sessions, a total of 3-6 sessions generally suffice to assess patient response in cases of lupus cerebritis or diffuse alveolar hemorrhage [[128]]. Some studies have evaluated longer therapies, though the efficacy and design are questionable.

Table 9. Recommendations for the use of plasmapheresis in the treatment of systemic lupus erythematosus during pregnancy [66]

Condition	Procedure	Recommendation	Category
Severe	PEX	Grade 2C	II
Nephritis	PEX	Grade 1B	IV

Schwartz J, Winters JL, Padmanabhan A, Balogun RA, Delaney M, Linenberger ML, Szczepiorkowski ZM, Williams ME, Wu Y, Shaz BH. Guidelines on the Use of Therapeutic Apheresis in Clinical Practice—Evidence-Based Approach from the Writing Committee of the American Society for Apheresis: The Sixth Special Issue. Journal of Clinical Apheresis 28:145–284 (2013).

Table 10. Plasmapheresis in systemic lupus erythematosus [66]

Volumen treated	1-1.5 TPV
Replacement Fluid	Albumin, plasma
Frequency	Lupus cerebrits or SLE with DAH: Daily or every other day; SLE other: 1-3 times per week

Despite the data obtained from the studies published to date, further information is needed to define a plasmapheresis protocol for the management of systemic lupus erythematosus.

Plasma Exchange in Other Disease Processes during Pregnancy

Gestational Pemphigoid

Gestational pemphigoid (GP) or gestational herpes is a pregnancy-induced autoimmune bullous dermatosis. Less frequent causes are estrogen and gestagen treatments or, in exceptional cases, trophoblastic tumors. It is a rare disease, with an incidence of between 1/2000 and 1/50,000 pregnancies [133]. The precise pathogenic mechanism is not clear, though the disease is believed to possibly have an autoimmune origin. A genetic predisposition to develop GP has been demonstrated – the condition being more common in women with certain major histocompatibility complex (MHC) class II antigens such as HLA-DR3, HLA-DR4 and HLA-B8 [134, 135].

Physiopathology

The autoimmune origin is suspected from the identification of linear deposits of complement fraction C3 and IgG in the basal membrane of the affected skin. It is believed that the aberrant expression of placental major histocompatibility complex class II antigens induces immunoallergic reactions between the maternal T lymphocytes and the antigens of the placental membrane - leading to the production of a pathological antiplacental IgG antibody [136, 137]. The latter in turn cross-reacts with an antigen that forms part of the hemidesmosomes of the dermoepidermal junction, known as BP-

AG2 (bullous pemphigoid antigen-2). This antigen is also present in the plasma membranes of the amniotic and umbilical cord cells, as well as in the chorial villi. The mentioned cross-reaction triggers the classical complement pathway, recruiting eosinophils and activating proteolytic enzymes that result in separation of the epidermis from the dermis [138, 139].

Clinical Manifestations

The main clinical manifestations of GP are intense itching and the appearance of skin lesions. Itching precedes or is concomitant to appearance of the skin lesions. The latter consist of urticarial papules or vesicles typically manifesting first in the periumbilical region [140]. The rash rapidly spreads outwards, with the final production of blisters. The lesions do not affect the face or scalp, and mucosal membrane involvement is exceptional. Gestational pemphigoid usually develops from the second or third trimester of pregnancy, though it can develop at any time during pregnancy and even during puerperium [141].

The disease usually resolves spontaneously, leaving no scars, within weeks or months after delivery. Recurrences in subsequent pregnancies are observed in 95% of all patients, and in such cases the condition is more severe and develops earlier [142].

The diagnosis is established from the skin biopsy and direct (DIF) and indirect immunofluorescence study (IIF). The biopsy sample shows subepidermal blisters associated to a dermoepidermal inflammatory infiltrate containing abundant eosinophils. Direct immunofluorescence confirms the diagnosis, revealing a dense linear and regular deposit of complement fraction C3 with or without IgG, along the dermoepidermal junction. Indirect immunofluorescence in turn detects the circulating pathological IgG autoantibody in 60-90% of all cases.

The maternal prognosis of GP is relatively good – the condition disappearing within 1-2 weeks after birth. However, the disease generally recurs in subsequent pregnancies, or with the use of oral contraceptives.

From the fetal viewpoint, GP may be associated to placental insufficiency that can lead to premature delivery, a low birth weight, and antepartum fetal death [143].

Treatment

The treatment of GP depends on the severity of the clinical manifestations.

During pregnancy, oral antihistamines, mild topical corticosteroids, emollients and oral prednisone are used.

During the first trimester antihistamines such as dexchlorpheniramine, dimetindene and clemastine are advised. Loratadine and cetirizine can be used in the second and third trimesters. Prednisone is regarded as the drug of choice, and is enzymatically inactivated in the placenta. The starting dose ranges from 0.5-2 mg/kg/day, depending on severity of the lesions. The maintenance dose should be the minimum effective dose, and should not exceed 10-15 mg/day during the first three months of pregnancy [144].

In severe cases, or after delivery, use has been made of immunosuppressants such as azathioprine or cyclosporin, and even immunomodulatory agents such as rituximab, plasmapheresis, or intravenous immunoglobulins.

Plasmapheresis is used to remove immunoglobulins or immune complexes from the bloodstream, and has been shown to be successful in antibody-mediated disorders such as gestational pemphigoid. There has been a report of a lack of response to plasmapheresis in a case of severe GP persisting for two years after delivery, in association with high-dose prednisone, azathioprine and dapsone [145]. However, a more recent report has described a case of severe GP in a 30-year-old pregnant woman treated with high-dose oral corticosteroids, with partial control, in which plasmapheresis yielded excellent results, with the performance of several prenatal and postnatal sessions [146]. Another case of success with plasmapheresis has been documented in a 40-year-old woman in week 20 of pregnancy, with rapid resolution of the itching and skin lesions [147]. In addition, no significant side effects have been seen.

Plasmapheresis as a therapeutic option in gestational pemphigoid appears to offer benefits, but should be reserved for serious cases that prove resistant to the usual treatments.

Acute Pancreatitis due to Hypertriglyceridemia

Hypertriglyceridemia (HTG) is the third leading cause of acute pancreatitis (AP), after alcohol and biliary lithiasis [148]. It reportedly accounts for 1-38% of all cases of AP, and for up to 56% of all cases of pancreatitis in pregnancy [149].

Hypertriglyceridemia is defined as fasting serum triglyceride levels of > 150 mg/dl. The condition is classified as follows:

- Mild: 150-199 mg/dl or 1.7-2.2 mmol/l
- Moderate: 200-999 mg/dl or 2.3-11.2 mmol/l
- Severe: 1000-1999 mg/dl or 11.2-22.4 mmol/l
- Very severe: > 2000 mg/dl or > 22.4 mmol/l [4]

Hypertriglyceridemia with levels of > 1000 mg/dl (> 11.2 mmol/l) [150] is considered to imply a risk of pancreatitis. The early detection of HTG associated to pancreatitis is extremely important in order to provide adequate treatment and prevent further episodes. Hypertriglyceridemia-induced pancreatitis is a serious complication of familial dyslipidemias. During pregnancy, hormonal influences in patients with familial hypertriglyceridemia can cause alterations in controlled lipid levels, producing susceptibility towards pancreatitis, and resulting in a significant increase in maternal-fetal morbidity.

Triglyceride (TG) levels of ≥ 1000 mg/dl increase the risk of acute pancreatitis (AP), though AP has also been reported in patients with lower TG levels. Hypertriglyceridemia in itself does not appear to be toxic. Rather, TG breakdown to toxic free fatty acids mediated by the action of pancreatic lipases is the cause of lipotoxicity in acute pancreatitis [151]. Thus, the severity of AP in patients with HTG depends both on the inflammatory response to AP, and on the damage caused by lipotoxicity secondary to the hydrolysis of triglycerides.

Primary Hypertriglyceridemia

According to the Frederickson classification [152], group I, IV and V dyslipidemias are associated with severe HTG, and these patients are susceptible to the development of AP [153].

Secondary Hypertriglyceridemia

A number of circumstances can increase the TG levels and lead to pancreatitis secondary to hypertriglyceridemia (PHTG) [154, 155]. Type 2 diabetes mellitus, and type 1 diabetes with diabetic ketoacidosis, can induce PHTG. Both hyperglycemia and HTG are probably related to a lack of insulin and to the effects of stress hormones. In these cases HTG responds to insulin therapy.

Alcohol can cause PHTG, though it is not clear whether alcohol does so directly or simply exacerbates underlying genetic hyperlipidemia [156]. Alcohol increases the serum triglyceride levels in a dose-dependent manner.

Hormone replacement therapy with estrogens [157] or tamoxifen [158] also increases triglyceride levels in serum. Hormone replacement therapy in women is not recommended when the serum triglyceride levels are > 500 mg/dl, due to an increased risk of PHTG.

It has been reported that pregnancy-induced HTG may be responsible for up to 56% of all cases of AP occurring during pregnancy.

The rise in estrogen levels during pregnancy induces an increase in the synthesis of very low density lipoproteins (VLDLs) in the liver [159, 160].

Human placental lactogen increases lipolysis in the adipose tissue and the free fatty acid levels in blood, facilitating the availability of metabolic substrates in the liver for triglyceride synthesis [161]. Lipoprotein lipase (LPL) activity is furthermore decreased during pregnancy [162]. The combination of these phenomena leads to an increased production of VLDLs; this, and the decrease in triglyceride clearance, results in a net increase in triglyceride levels. In healthy patients the triglyceride levels usually do not exceed 300 mg/dl (3.3 mmol/l). This serum triglyceride concentration is not enough to produce pancreatitis. However, in patients with dyslipidemic disorders such as type I, IV and V familial hyperlipidemia syndrome, this increase in VLDL synthesis is not controlled and gives rise to severe hypertriglyceridemia, with a significant increase in the risk of AP and in maternal-fetal morbidity.

The initial presentation of PHTG is similar to that of acute pancreatitis of other causes. Abdominal pain, nausea and vomiting are the main symptoms.

Laboratory tests to determine amylase, GOT, GPT, GGT, alkaline phosphatase, total bilirubin, glucose, urea/blood urea nitrogen (BUN), creatinine, calcium, sodium and potassium are required, together with a blood count.

Excess serum triglycerides can produce a false decrease in blood amylase levels. In this case lipase may be useful in clinical conditions that have developed over several days, since its clearance is slower than that of amylase. Amylase levels in urine also can be measured, and are found to be increased in patients with pancreatitis.

Treatment

A first step in patients with hypertriglyceridemia should be the adoption of preventive measures, with control of the triglyceride levels [163].

In view of the teratogenic effects associated with the use of fibrates, alternative strategies are required during pregnancy [164] for the treatment of hypertriglyceridemia. Several reports of PHTG in pregnancy have described the use of apheresis [165, 166], intravenous glucose and insulin [167], intravenous heparin [168], and low fat diets. Successful control of HTG, with the delivery of a healthy infant, was recorded in all cases.

In patients with severe PHTG, apheresis appears to be able to reduce mortality [169, 170]. Therapeutic plasma exchange (PEX) is the treatment of choice for PHTG, due to the possibility of triglyceride-induced filter obstruction [171].

The main concerns referred to apheresis include the cost and availability of the technique. After a treatment cycle, if the serum triglyceride levels are < 500 mg/dl, no further apheresis cycles are performed. Apheresis is reintroduced if the triglyceride levels are subsequently seen to increase again. The early introduction of apheresis is very likely to offer beneficial effects. Apheresis is generally started as soon as possible. Successful PEX for preventing PHTG in the case of serum triglyceride levels of > 1000 mg/dl has also been described, avoiding the development of AP during pregnancy and delivering a healthy infant [172].

Insulin

If apheresis is not available, if the patient shows poor tolerance of apheresis, or if the serum glucose levels exceed 500 mg/dl, intravenous insulin is used. Insulin reduces the serum triglyceride levels, improving the activity of lipoprotein lipase (LPL), an enzyme that accelerates the metabolization of VLDLs and chylomicrons to glycerol and free fatty acids [173].

Insulin also inhibits a hormone-sensitive lipase in the adipocytes that is crucial for degrading triglycerides within the adipose cells, with fatty acid release into the bloodstream.

Intravenous insulin administration is preferred to subcutaneous injection in cases of severe PHTG [174].

Capillary blood glucose monitoring is advised every four hours, with the measurement of triglyceride levels every 12-24 hours, adjusting the insulin dosage accordingly. It is advisable to discontinue intravenous insulin when the triglyceride levels drop to below 500 mg/dl.

Heparin

The role of heparin is controversial. It stimulates the release of endothelial lipoprotein lipase into the bloodstream [175], and has been used without insulin in the management of hypertriglyceridemia [176].

Despite the reported success of intravenous heparin in combination with insulin in the management of hypertriglyceridemia, heparin use to treat PHTG has been criticized. The benefits of heparin are temporary and result in faster depletion of the endothelial lipoprotein lipase reserves, giving rise to an increase in chylomicron concentration [177]. On the other hand, heparin increases the risk of bleeding.

Acute pancreatitis secondary to hypertriglyceridemia is a serious disease, particularly during pregnancy. Of all the available treatment modalities, plasmapheresis appears to be the most effective and safe option during pregnancy for both treating and preventing acute pancreatitis.

Acute Gravidic Liver Steatosis

Acute gravidic liver steatosis (AGLS) is characterized by microvesicular steatosis of the liver cells, and is an inherent disorder of human pregnancy. The condition is of sudden onset and typically manifests during the third trimester. The disease was first described in 1940 [178], and was believed to be inevitably fatal, progressing to fulminant liver failure and coagulation disorders with or without hepatic encephalopathy in women with no previous liver disease. However, it is now known that an early diagnosis, together with the termination of pregnancy, results in a spectacularly improved prognosis [179].

Acute gravidic liver steatosis is a rare condition with an approximate incidence of 1/7000 - 1/20,000 deliveries [180, 181].

The underlying cause remains unknown, though fetal or maternal functional deficits in certain mitochondrial long-chain fatty acid oxidation enzymes have been described in some cases as a possible explanation for the disorder [182].

The disease is always present prior to delivery but is not always diagnosed. The most common initial symptoms are nausea and vomiting (in 75% of the cases), abdominal pain (mainly epigastric pain)(50%), anorexia and jaundice. Signs of preeclampsia have been described at onset or during the course of the disease [183].

Pregnant women with AGLS present hypertransaminasemia. Hyperbilirubinemia and leukocytosis are usually also observed. Patients with severe AGLS also show increased urea, prolonged prothrombin time and hypoglycemia secondary to liver failure. Acute renal failure, thrombocytopenia and hyperuricemia have often been reported.

Physiopathology

The association of cases of AGLS to fetal deficiency of one of the enzymes responsible for the mitochondrial beta-oxidation of fatty acids, long-chain 3-hydroxyacyl-CoA-dehydrogenase (LCHAD), suggests that some women and their fetuses could have a hereditary beta-oxidation enzyme defect predisposing the mother to AGLS [184, 185]. LCHAD catalyzes the third step of fatty acid beta-oxidation at mitochondrial level. The accumulation of long-chain 3-hydroxyacyl metabolites produced by the fetus or placenta is hepatotoxic, and could be the cause of liver damage [186, 187]. Nevertheless, some authors have not been able to confirm this association to LCHAD [188, 189]. A possible explanation would be that only specific genetic deficiencies associated to LCHAD lead to an increased risk of AGLS [190]. Another possible explanation for the absence of detected LCHAD mutations could be the existence of other fatty acid beta-oxidation deficiencies associated to AGLS [191].

Diagnosis

In addition to the clinical suspicion of AGLS, the diagnosis is based on the detection of initial laboratory test alterations such as hypertransaminasemia (under 25 times the normal value) and hyperuricemia with bilirubinemia, in addition to coagulation factors, serum creatinine and leukocyte values that are normal or almost normal in the early stage of the disease [192]. Imaging techniques such as ultrasound or abdominal computed axial tomography usually do not offer much information at the time of diagnosis. However, comparison of the images with those obtained after delivery may then reveal the existence of steatosis [193].

The diagnosis may be established by applying the criteria of Swansea, with confirmation of AGLS in the presence of at least 6 of the following symptoms: nausea, abdominal pain, polydipsia/polyuria, encephalopathy, hypoglycemia, hyperuricemia, leukocytosis, ascites, transaminase elevation, hyperbilirubinemia, hyperuricemia, renal failure, coagulopathy (decrease in prothrombin time), microvascular steatosis at liver biopsy, and metabolic acidosis [194].

Histological study of the liver biopsy confirms the diagnosis, revealing characteristic microvesicular steatosis infiltrating the centrilobular hepatocytes, with no change in the centralized position of the cell nucleus [195]. However, liver biopsy is an invasive procedure, and is therefore not frequently performed. Precautions are moreover required when performing a liver biopsy during pregnancy, reserving the technique for cases of diagnostic doubt and when needing to postpone the termination of pregnancy.

The differential diagnosis of AGLS is mainly established with HELLP syndrome (hemophilic anemia, hypertransaminasemia and thrombocytopenia).

Treatment

There is no specific medical treatment for AGLS. The first therapeutic option is the termination of pregnancy, often on an emergency basis, after stabilization of the patient.

Maternal stabilization is achieved through blood glucose control, the intravenous administration of glucose, and coagulopathy control with the infusion of fresh frozen plasma (FFP), red cell concentrates or platelets.

Plasmapheresis is a recently introduced management option. In theory, plasmapheresis allows the elimination of endotoxins, bilirubin, urea and inflammatory cytokines from blood – these processes being carried out by the liver cells under physiological conditions [196]. In addition, the administration of large volumes of FFP by plasmapheresis allows us to improve the coagulation parameters and renal function.

A recent article has reported three cases of successful treatment with plasmapheresis [197]. The first case corresponded to a 22-year-old woman in her first pregnancy who developed renal and liver failure, coagulopathy and respiratory failure requiring mechanical ventilation, with a diagnosis of AGLS in week 37 of pregnancy. Pregnancy was terminated as a first measure, and plasmapheresis with the provision of FFP was decided after clinical worsening. Twenty-two plasmapheresis sessions were required to normalize the biological parameters. The next case corresponded to a 23-year-old woman in week 37 of her second pregnancy who was diagnosed with AGLS.

After fetal extraction, four plasmapheresis sessions were carried out until clinical and laboratory test improvement was achieved. The third case corresponded to a 23-year-old woman in week 36 of her first pregnancy. After pregnancy termination and three plasmapheresis sessions, all the biological parameters returned to normal.

Another study assessing the therapeutic effects of plasmapheresis in 39 patients with AGLS likewise reported favorable results. There were no serious side effects or situations leading to treatment discontinuation. Both liver and kidney function improved significantly after treatment with plasmapheresis. Furthermore, the authors found that the sooner treatment was started, the lesser the need to repeat plasmapheresis [198].

As a result, plasmapheresis is regarded as a good therapeutic option, particularly in severe AGLS.

Most patients with severe disease recover without liver sequelae [199], though there have been reports of important morbidity and mortality.

The recurrence risk is not known. Subsequent pregnancies are therefore considered to be high risk situations requiring adequate monitorization.

Authors do not have any competing interest to declare

REFERENCES

[1] Eser B, Guven M, Unol A, Coskun R, Altuntas F, Sungur M, Serin IS, et al. The role of plasma exchange in the HELLP síndrome. *Clin. Appl. Thromb. Hemost.* 2005;11:2:11-7.

[2] Kambic, H. E. and Nosé, Y. (1997), Historical Perspective on Plasmapheresis. *Therapeutic Apheresis*, 1: 83–108. doi: 10.1111/j.1744-9987.1997.

[3] Nakanishi T, Suzuki N, Kuragano T, Nagasawa Y, Hasuike Y. Current topics intherapeutic plasmapheresis. *Clin. Exp. Nephrol.* 2013.

[4] Shariatmadar et al. Effect of plasma Exchange on cytokines measured by multianalyte bead array in thrombotic thrombocyttopenic purpura. *Am. J. Hematol.* 2005;79:83-88.

[5] Winters JL. Plasma Exchange: concepts, mecanisms and an overview of the American Society for Apheresis guidelines. *Hematology*. 2012;8:1:7-12.

[6] Kaplan AA. Toward the rational prescription of thepauteic plasma Exchange: the kinetics of inmunoglobulin removal. *Semin. Dial.* 1992; 5:227-9.

[7] Anaya-Fernandez lomana F. Complicaciones aféresis terapéutica. En: Anaya-Fernandez lomana F. Manual de aféresis terapéutica basada en la evidencía. Barcelona: Ed Nefrología de la Sociedad Española de Nefrología; 2012. p141-149.

[8] Kaplan A. Therapeutic plasma Exchange: A technical an operational review. *Journal of clinical apheresis* 2013; 28: DOI: 10.1002/jca.21257.

[9] Shemin D, Briggs D, Greenan M. Complications of therapeutic plasma Exchange: A prospective study of 1727 cases. *Journal of clinical apheresis* 2007; 22:270-276.

[10] Miller D, Kaye JA, Shea K, et al. Incidence of Thrombotic Thrombocytopenic Purpura/Hemolytic Uremic Syndrome. *Epidemiology* 2004; 15: 208-215.

[11] Egerman RS, Witlin AG, Friedman SA, et al. Thrombotic thrombocytopenic purpura and hemolytic uremic syndrome in pregnancy: review of 11 cases. *Am. J. Obstet. Gynecol.* 1996; 175: 950–956.

[12] Moatti-Cohen M, Garrec C, Wolf M, et al. Unexpected frequency of Upshaw-Schulman syndrome in pregnancy-onset thrombotic thrombocytopenic purpura. *Blood* 2012; 119: 5888-5897.

[13] Ezra Y, Rose M, Eldor A. Therapy and prevention of thrombotic thrombocytopenic purpura during pregnancy: A clinical study of 16 pregnancies. *Am. J. Hematol.* 1996; 51:1- 6.

[14] Battaglioli T, Valsecchi C, Lavoretano S, Mannucci PM, Peyvandi F, Palla R: Risk factors for recurrence of thrombotic thrombocytopenic purpura. *Blood* 2006; 108:11.

[15] Scully M, Yarranton H, Liesner R, et al. Regional United Kingdom TTP registry: correlation with laboratory ADAMTS13 analysis and clinical fea-tures. *Br. J. Haematol.* 2008;142(5):819-826.

[16] Fujimura Y, Matsumoto M. Registry of 919 pa- tients with thrombotic microangiopathies across Japan: database of Nara medical university dur- ing 1998-2008. *Intern. Med.* 2010; 49(1):7-15.

[17] Peyvandi F, Lavoretano S, Palla R, et al. ADAMTS 13 and anti-ADAMTS 13 antibodies as markers for recurrence of acquired thrombotic thrombocytopenic purpura during remission. *Haematologica* 2008; 93: 232-239.

[18] DÁngelo A, Fattorini A, Crippa L. Thrombotic microangiopathy in pregnancy. *Thrombosis research* 2009; 123 (Suppl): 556-562.
[19] Natelson EA, White D. Recurrent thrombotic thrombocytopenic purpura in early pregnancy: Effect of uterine evacuation. *Obstet. Gynecol.* 1985; 66:45s 54s.
[20] Trisolini SM, Capria S, Gozzer M, et al. Thrombotic thrombocytopenic purpura in the first trimester and successful pregnancy. *Ann. Hematol.* 2009; 88:287–289.
[21] Martin JN, Bailey A, Rehberg JF, et al. Thrombotic thrombocytopenic purpura in 166 pregnancies-2006. *American Journal of Obstetrics and Gynecology* 2008; 199:98-104.
[22] George JN. The association of pregnancy with thrombotic thromcytopenic purpura-hemolyticuremic syndrome. *Curr. Opin. Hematol.* 2003, 10:339–344.
[23] Moschovitz E. Hyaline thrombosis of the terminal arterioles and capilliaries: a a hitherto undiscribed disease. *Proc. NY Pathol. Soc.* 1924; 24.21-4.
[24] Miner PF, Nutt RL, Thomas ME. Thrombotic thrombocytopenic purpura occurring during pregnancy. *Am. J. Obstet. Gynecol.* 1955; 70:611-617.
[25] Lotta LA, Lombardi R, MarianiM, et al. Platelet reactive conformation and multimeric pattern of von Willebrand factor in acquired thrombotic thrombocytopenic purpura during acute disease and remission. *J. Thromb. Haemost.* 2011; 9:1744-51.
[26] Moake JL, Rudy CK, Troll JH, Weinstein MJ, Colamino NM, Azocar J, et al. Unusually large plasma factor VIII: vonWillebrand factor multimers in chronic relapsing thrombotic thrombocytopenic purpura. *N. Eng. J. Med.* 1982; 307;1432-1435.
[27] Moake JL, Turner NA, Stathopoulos NA, Nolasco LH, Hellums JD. Involvement of large plasma von Willebrand factor multimers and usually large VWF forms derived from endotelial cells in shear stress-induced platelet aggregation. *J. Clin. Invest.* 1986; 78: 1456-1461.
[28] Moake JL. Thrombotic microangiopathies. *N. Engl. J. Med.* 2002; 347: 589-600.
[29] Camilleri RS, Scully M, Thomas M, Mackie IJ, Liesner R, Chen WJ, Manns K, Machin SJ. A phenotype-genotype correlation of ADAMTS13 mutations in congenital thrombotic thrombocytopenic purpura patients treated in the United Kingdom. *J. Thromb. Haemost.* 2012;10(9):1792-801.

[30] Levy GA, Nichols WC, Lian EC, Foroud T, McClintick JN, McGee BM, Yang AY, Siemieniak DR, Stark KR, Gruppo R, Sarode R, Shurin SB, Chandrasekaran V, Stabler SP, Sabio H, Bouhassira EE, Upshaw JD Jr, Ginsburg D, Tsai HM: Mutations in a member of the ADAMTS gene family cause thrombotic thrombocytopenic purpura. *Nature* 2001, 413:488-494.

[31] Murrin RJA, Murray JA. Thrombotic Thrombocytopenic purpura: aetiology, pathophysiology and treatment. *Blood Reviews*. 200; 20:51-60.

[32] Gernesheimer T, james AH, Stasi R. How I treat thrombocytopenia in pregnancy. *Blood* 2013; 121:38-47.

[33] Scully M, Starke R, Lee R: Successful management of pregnancy in women with a history of thrombotic thrombocytopenic purpura. *Blood Coagul. Fibrinolysis* 2006, 17:459-463.

[34] Ridolfi RL, Bell WR. Thrombotic thrombocytopenic purpura. Report of 25 cases and review of the iterature. *Medicine* (Baltimore) 1981; 60(6):413-28.

[35] George JN. How I treat patients with thrombotic thrombocytopenic purpura: 2010. *Blood* 2010; 116:4060-4069.

[36] Rock GA, Shumak KH, Buskard NA, et al. Com- parison of plasma exchange with plasma infusion in the treatment of thrombotic thrombocytopenic purpura. *N. Engl. J. Med.* 1991;3 25(6):393-397.

[37] Coppo P, Veyradier A. Current management and therapeutical perspectives in thrombotic thrombocytopenic purpura. *Presse Med.* 2012; 41:163-176.

[38] Bell WR, Braine HG, Ness PM, Kickler TS. Improved survival in thrombotic thrombocytopenic purpura- hemolytic uremic syndrome. Clinical experience in 108 patients. *N. Engl. J. Med.* 1991; 325(6):398-403.

[39] Balduini CL, Gugliotta L, Luppi M, Laurenti L, Klersy C, Pieresca C et al. High versus standard dose methylprednisolone in the acute phase of idiopathic thrombotic thrombocytopenic purpura: a randomized study. *Ann. Hematol.* 2010; 89(6):591-6.

[40] Scully M, Hunt BJ, Benjamin S, Liesner R, et al. Guidelines on the diagnosis and management of thrombotic thrombocytopenic purpura and other thrombotic microangiopathies. *British Journal of Haematology* 2012, 158, 323–335.

[41] Swisher KK, Terrell DR, Vesely SK, Kremer Hovinga JA, Lammle B, George JN. Clinical outcomes after latelet transfusions in patients with thrombotic thrombocytopenic purpura. *Transfusion* 2009;49(5):873-87.

[42] Ojeda-Uribe M, Federici L, Wolf M, Coppo P, Veyradler A: Successful long-term rituximab maintenance for a relapsing patient with idiopathic thrombotic thrombocytopenic purpura. *Transfusion* 2010; 50:733-735.

[43] Caramazza D, Quintini G, Abbene I, Coco LL, Malato A, Di Trapani R et al. Rituximab for managing relapsing or refractory patients with idiopathic thrombotic thrombocytopenic purpura–haemolytic uraemic syndrome. *Blood Transfus*. 2010; 8(3):203-10.

[44] Scully M, McDonald V, Cavenagh J, Hunt BJ, Longair I, Cohen H et al. A phase II study of the safety and efficacy of rituximab with plasma exchange in acute acquired thrombotic thrombocytopenic purpura. *Blood* 2011; 118(7):1746-53.

[45] Ojeda-Uribe M, Afif N, Dahan E, Sparsa L, Haby C, Sibilia J, Ternant D, Ardizzone M. Exposure to abatacept or rituximab in the first trimester of pregnancy in three women with autoimmune diseases. *Clin. Rheumatol.* 2013; 32(5):695-700.

[46] Dashe JS, Ramin SM, Cunningham FG. The long-term consequences of thrombotic microangiopathy thrombotic thrombocutopenic purpura and haemolytic uremic syndrome) in pregnancy. *Obstet. Gynecol.* 1998; 91:662–668.

[47] Proia A, Paesano R, Torcia F, Annino L, Capria S, Ferrari A, Ferrazza G, Pacifici E, Pantalissi A, Meloni G: Thrombotic thrombocytopenic purpura and pregnancy: a case report and a review of the literature. *Ann. Hematol.* 2002; 81:210-214.

[48] Weiner CP. Thrombotic microangiopathy in pregnancy and in the postpartum period. *Sem. Hematol*. 1987; 24:119–129.

[49] Proia A, Paesano R, Torcia F, Annino L, Capria S, Ferrari A, Ferrazza G, Pacifici E, Pantalissi A, Meloni G: Thrombotic thrombocytopenic purpura and pregnancy: a case report and a review of the literature. *Ann. Hematol.* 2002, 81:210-214.

[50] Shamseddine A, Chehal A, Salem Z, et al. Thrombotic Thrombocytopenic Purpura and Pregnancy: Report of four cases and literatura review. *Journal of clinical Apheresis* 2004; 19:5-10.

[51] González-Mesa E, Narbona I, Blasco M, Cohen I. *Journal of Medical Case Reports* 2013, 7:119.

[52] Plauché WC. Myasthenia gravis. *Clin. Obstet. Gynecol*. 1983; 26:592-604.

[53] Plauche WC. Myasthenia gravis in mothers and their newborns. *Clin. Obstet. Gynecol.* 1991; 34:82–99.

[54] Ciafaloni E, Massey J. Myasthenia gravis and pregnancy. *Neurol. Clin.* 2004; 22:771-782.

[55] Hoch W, McConville J, Helms S, Newsome-Davis J, Melms A, Vincent A. Autoantibodies to the receptor tyrosine kinase MuSK in patients with myasthenia gravis without acetylcholine receptor antibodies. *Nat. Med.* 2001;7:365–8.

[56] Zhang B, Tzartos JS, Belimezi M, Ragheb S, Bealmear B, Lewis RA, et al. Autoanti- bodies to lipoprotein-related protein 4 in patients with double-seronegative myasthenia gravis. *Arch. Neurol.* 2012;69:445–51.

[57] Ferrero S, Pretta S, Nicoletti A, Petrera P, Ragni N. Myasthenia gravis: management issues during pregnancy. *Eur. J. Obstet. Gynecol. Reprod. Biol.* 2005; 121:129-38.

[58] Watson WJ, Katz VL, Bowes WA. Plasmapheresis during pregnancy. *Obstet. Gynecol.* 1984; 76:451–7.

[59] Ebadi H, Barth D, Bril V. Safety of plasma exchange therapy in patients with myasthenia gravis. *Muscle Nerve* Apr 2013;47:510–4.

[60] Samuels P, Pfeifer SM. Autoimmune diseases in pregnancy. The obstetrician's view. *Rheum. Dis. Clin. North Am.* 1989;15:307–22.

[61] Armenti VT, Moritz MJ, Davison JM. Drug safety issues in pregnancy following transplantation and immunosuppression: effects and outcomes. *Drug Saf.* 1998;19:219–32.

[62] Lewis RA. Myasthenia gravis: New therapeutic approaches based on pathophysiology. *Journal of the Neurological Sciences* 333 (2013) 93–98.

[63] Carr SR, Gilchrist JM, Abeulo DN, Clark D. Treatment of antenatal myasthenia gravis. *Obstet. Gynaecol.* 1991;78:485–9.

[64] Mari G, Deter RL, Carpenter RL, et al. Noninvasive Diagnosis by Doppler Ultrasonography of Fetal Anemia Due to Maternal Red-Cell Alloimmunization. *N. Engl. J. Med.* 2000; 342:9-14.

[65] American College of Obstetricians and Gynecologists. Guidelines for perinatal care. 6th ed. Washington, DC: American College of Obstetricians and Gynecologists; 2007: 104.

[66] Schawartz J, Winters JL, Padmanabhan A, Balogun RA, Delaney M, Linenberger ML, et al. Guidelines on theOse of Therapeutic Apheresis in Clinical Practice. Evidence-Based Approach from the Writing Committee of the American Society for Apheresis: The Sixth Special Issue. *Journal of Clinical Apheresis*. 2013; 28:145-284.

[67] Ruma MS, Moise KJ Jr, Kim E, Murtha AP, Prutsman WJ, Hassan SS, Lubarsky SL. Combined plasmapheresis and intravenous immune globulin for the treatment of severe maternal red cellalloimmunization. *Am. J. Obstet. Gynecol.* 2007 Feb;196(2):138.

[68] Palfi M, Hildén JO, Matthiesen L, Selbing A, Berlin G. A case of severe Rh (D) alloimmunization treated by intensive plasma exchange and high-dose intravenous immunoglobulin. *Transfus. Apher. Sci.* 2006 Oct; 35(2):131-6. Epub 2006 Oct 11.

[69] Novak DJ, Tyler LN, Reddy RL, Barsoom MJ. Plasmapheresis and intravenous immune globulin for the treatment of D alloimmunization in pregnancy. *J. Clin. Apher.* 2008;23(6):183-5.

[70] Isojima S, Hisano M, Suzuki T, Sago H, Murashima A, Yamaguchi K. Early plasmapheresis followed by high-dose γ-globulin treatment saved a severely Rho-incompatible pregnancy. *J. Clin. Apher.* 2011;26(4): 216-8.

[71] Fernández-Jiménez MC, Jiménez-Marco MT, Hernández D, González A, Omeñaca F, de la Cámara C. Treatment with plasmapheresis and intravenous immunoglobulin in pregnancies complicated with anti-PP1Pk or anti-K immunization: a report of two patients. *Vox. Sang.* 2001 Feb;80(2):117-20.

[72] Levine JS, Branch DW, Rauch J. The antiphospholipid syndrome. *N. Engl. J. Med.* 2002 Mar 7; 346(10):752-63.

[73] Cervera R, Piette JC, Font J, et al. Antiphospholipid syndrome: clinical and immunologic manifestations and patterns of disease expression in a cohort of 1,000 patients. *Arthritis Rheum.* 2002; 46: 1019-1027.

[74] Asherson RA, Cervera R, Font J. Multiorgan thrombotic disorders in systemic lupus erythematosus: a common link? *Lupus.* 1992 Aug; 1(4):199-203.

[75] Lim W. Antiphospholipid syndrome. *Hematology Am. Soc. Hematol. Educ. Program.* 2013;2013:675-80.

[76] Asherson RA, Cervera R, de Groot PG, Erkan D, Boffa MC, Piette JC, et al. Catastrophic antiphospholipid syndrome: international consensus statement on classification criteria and treatment guidelines. *Lupus.* 2003;12(7):530-4.

[77] Cohen D, Berger SP, Steup-Beekman GM, Bloemenkamp KW, Bajema IM. Diagnosis and management of the antiphospholipid syndrome. *BMJ.* 2010;340:2541.

[78] Pengo V, Ruffatti A, Legnani C, Gresele P, Barcellona D, Erba N, et al. Clinical course of high risk patients diagnosed with antiphospholipid syndrome (APS). *J. Thromb. Haemost.* 2010; 8: 237–42.

[79] Meroni PL, Gerosa M, Raschi E, Scurati S, Grossi C, Borghi MO. Updating on the pathogenic mechanisms 5 of the antiphos-pholipid antibodies-associated pregnancy loss. *Clin. Rev. Allergy Immunol.* 2008; 34:332–7.

[80] Miyakis S, Lockshin MD, Atsumi T, Branch DW, Brey RL, Cervera R, et al. International consensus statement on an update of the classification criteria for definite antiphospholipid syndrome (APS). *J. Thromb. Haemost.* 2006 Feb;4(2):295-306.

[81] Van den Boogaard E, Hermens RP, Franssen AM, et al. Recurrent miscarriage: do professionals adhere to their guidelines. *Hum. Reprod.* 2013; 28: 2898-2904.

[82] Ruffatti A, Calligaro A, Hoxha A, et al. Laboratory and clinical features of pregnant women with antiphospholipid syndrome and neonatal outcome. *Arthritis Care Res.* 2010; 62: 302-307.

[83] Cervera R, Serrano R, Pons-Estel GJ, Ceberio-Hualde L, Shoenfeld Y. et al. Morbidity and mortality in the antiphospholipid syndrome during a 10-year period: a multicentre prospective study of 1000 patients. *Ann. Rheum. Dis.* 2014 Jan 24.

[84] Hanouna G, Morel N, Le Thi Huong D, et al. Catastrophic antiphospholipid syndrome and pregnancy: an experience of 13 cases. *Rheumatology* (Oxford). 2013; 52: 1635-1641.

[85] Pels SG, Paidas MJ. Microangiopathic Disorders in Pregnancy. *Hematol. Oncol. Clin. N. Am.* 2011; 25: 311-322.

[86] Task Force on hypertension in Pregnancy. The American College of Obstetricians and Gynecologists. Hypertension in Pregnancy. Practice Guideline WQ 244. ISBN 978-1-934984-28-4.

[87] Martin JN, Blake PG, Perry KG, McCaul JF, Hess LW, Martin RW. The natural history of HELLP síndrome: patterns of disease progression and regression. *American Journal Obstetrics and Gynecology* 1991; 164: 1500-1513.

[88] Danowski A, Rego J, Kakehasi AM, et al. Guidelines for the treatment of antiphospholipid syndrome. *Rev. Bras. Reumatol.* 2013; 53: 184-192.

[89] Bergrem A, Jacobsen EM, Skjeldestad FE, Jacobsen AF, Skogstad M, Sandset PM. The association of antiphospholipid antibodies with pregnancy-related fi rst time venous thrombosis – a populationbased case-control study. *Thromb. Res.* 2010;125(5):e222-7.

[90] Quenby S, Farquharson RG, Dawood F, Hughes AM, Topping J. Recurrent miscarriage and long-term thrombosis risk: a case-control study. *Hum. Reprod.* 2005;20(6):1729-32.

[91] Marchetti T, Cohen M, Gris JC, de Moerloose P. Diagnosis and management of obstetrical antiphospholipid syndrome: where do we stand? *Pol. Arch. Med. Wewn.* 2013 Dec 24;123(12):713-20.

[92] Alijotas-Reig J. Treatment of refractory obstetric antiphospholipid syndrome: the state of the art and new trends in the therapeutic management. *Lupus.* 2013; 22: 6-17.

[93] Schawartz J, Winters JL, Padmanabhan A, Balogun RA, Delaney M, Linenberger ML, et al. Guidelines on theOse of Therapeutic Apheresis in Clinical Practice. Evidence-Based Approach from the Writing Committee of the American Society for Apheresis: The Sixth Special Issue. *Journal of Clinical Apheresis.* 2013; 28:145-284.

[94] Bucciarelli S, Espinosa G, Cervera R, et al. Mortality in the catastrophic antiphospholipid syndrome: causes of death and prognostic factors in a series of 250 patients. *Arthritis Rheum.* 2006; 54:2568.

[95] Bontadi A, Ruffatti A, Marson P, Tison T, Tonello M, Hoxha A, De Silvestro G, Punzi L. Plasma exchange and immunoadsorption effectively remove antiphospholipid antibodies in pregnant patients with antiphospholipid syndrome. *J. Clin. Apher.* 2012;27(4):200-4.

[96] El-Haieg DO, Zanati MF, El-Foual FM. Plasmapheresis and pregnancy outcome in patients with antiphospholipid syndrome. *Int. J. Gynaecol. Obstet.* 2007 Dec;99(3):236-41. Epub 2007 Sep 25.

[97] Ruffatti A, Marson P, Pengo V, Favaro M, Tonello M, Bortolati M, Minucci D, De Silvestro G. Plasma exchange in the management of high risk pregnant patients with primary antiphospholipid syndrome. A report of 9 cases and a review of the literature. *Autoimmun. Rev.* 2007 Jan; 6(3):196-202.

[98] Ruiz-Irastorza G, Khamashta MA. Lupus and pregnancy: integrating clues from the bench and bedside. *Eur. J. Clin. Invest.* 2011 Jun; 41(6): 672-8.

[99] D'Cruz DP, Khamashta MA, Hughes GR. Systemic lupus erythematosus. *Lancet* 2007; 369: 587 - 96.

[100] Zen M, Ghirardello A, Iaccarino L et al. Hormones, immune response, and pregnancy in healthy women and SLE patients. *Swiss Med. Wkly.* 2010 Apr 3;140(13-14):187-201.

[101] Fatemi A, Fard RM, Sayedbonakdar Z et al. The role of lupus nephritis in development of adverse maternal and fetal outcomes during pregnancy. *Int. J. Prev. Med.* 2013 Sep;4(9):1004-10.

[102] Patel T, Fenves A, Colbert G. The de novo diagnosis of systemic lupus erithematosus and lupus nephritis during pregnancy. *Proc.* (Bayl Univ Med Cent). 2012 Apr;25(2):129-31.

[103] Clowse ME. Lupus activity in pregnancy. *Rheum. Dis. Clin. North Am.* 3(2007) 237-252.

[104] Ateka-Barrutia O, Khamashta MA. The challenge of pregnancy for patients with SLE. *Lupus.* 2013 Oct;22(12):1295-308.

[105] Lozza I, Cianci S, Di Natale A, Garofalo G, Giacobbe AM, Giorgio E, De Oronzo MA, Politi S. Update on systemic lupus erythematosus pregnancy. *Journal of Prenatal Medicine* 2010; 4 (4): 67-73.

[106] Baer AN, Witter FR, Petri M. Lupus and pregnancy. *Obstet. Gynecol. Surv.* 2011 Oct;66(10):639-53.

[107] Rahman FZ, Rahman J, Al-Suleiman et al. Pregnancy outcome in lupus nephropathy. *Arch. Gynecol. Obstet.* 2005; 271(3): 222-6.

[108] Yan Yuen S, Krizov, A, Ouimet JM et al. pregnancy outcome in systemic lupus erythemmatosus is improving: results from a case control study and literature review. *Open Rheumatol. J.* 2008; 2: 89-98.

[109] Clowse ME, Magder LS, Witter F, Petri M. The impact of increased lupus activity on obstetric outcomes. *Arthritis Rheum.* 2005 Feb; 52(2):514-21.

[110] Ostensen M, Clowse M. Pathogenesis of pregnancy complications in systemic lupus erythematosus. *Curr. Opin. Rheumatol.* 2013 Sep; 25(5):591-6.

[111] CLowse ME, Jamison M, Myers E et al. A national study of the complications of lupus in pregnancy. *Am. J. Obstet. Gyneacol.* 2008; 199 (2):127.e1-6.

[112] Shahian M, Khosravi A, Anbardar MH. Earlycholestasis in neonatal lupuserythematosus. *Ann. Saudi Med.* 2011 Jan-Feb;31(1):80-2.

[113] Hornberger LK, Al Rajaa N. Spectrum of cardiac involvement in neonatal lupus. *Scand. J. Immunol.* 2010 Sep;72(3):189-97.

[114] Brucato A, Previtali E, Ramoni V et al. Arrhythmias presenting in neonatal lupus. *Scand. J. Immunol.* 2010 Sep;72(3):198-204.

[115] Silverman E, Jaeggi E. Non-cardiac manifestations of neonatal lupus erythematosus. *Scand. J. Immunol.* 2010 Sep;72(3):223-5.

[116] Shahian M, Khosravi A, Anbardar MH. Early cholestasis in neonatal lupus erythematosus. *Ann. Saudi Med.* 2011 Jan-Feb;31(1):80-2.

[117] Levy RA, Vilela VS, Cataldo MJ et al. Hydroxychloroquine (HCQ) in lupuspregnancy: double-blind and placebo-controlled study. *Lupus.* 2001;10(6):401-4.

[118] Clowse ME, Magder L, Witter F et al. Hydroxychloroquine in lupuspregnancy. *Arthritis Rheum.* 2006 Nov;54(11):3640-7.

[119] Costedoat-Chalumeau N, Amoura Z, Duhaut P et al. Safety of hydroxychloroquine in pregnant patients with connective tissue diseases: a study of one hundred thirty-three cases compared with a control group. *Arthritis Rheum.* 2003 Nov;48(11):3207-11.

[120] Ostensen M. Diseasespecificproblemsrelated to drugtherapy in pregnancy. *Lupus.* 2004;13(9):746-50.

[121] Barbhaiya M, Bermas BL. Evaluation and management of systemic lupus erythematosus and rheumatoid arthritis during pregnancy. *Clin. Immunol.* 2013 Nov;149(2):225-35.

[122] Goldstein LH, Dolinsky G, Greenberg R et al. Pregnancyoutcome of womenexposed to azathioprine during pregnancy. *Birth Defects Res. A Clin. Mol. Teratol.* 2007 Oct;79(10):696-701.

[123] Clowse ME, Magder L, Petri M. Cyclophosphamide for lupus during pregnancy. *Lupus.* 2005;14(8):593-7.

[124] Ostensen M, Khamashta M, Lockshin M et al. Antyinflammatory and inmunosupresive drugs and reproduction. *Arthritis Res. Ther.* 8 (2006) 209.

[125] Chakravarty EF, Murray ER, Kelman A et al. Pregnancy outcomes after maternal exposure to rituximab. *Blood.* 2011 Feb 3;117(5):1499-506.

[126] Samson M, Audia S, Leguy V, Berthier S, Janikashvili N, Martin L et al. Haemolytic-uraemic síndrome during severe lupus nephritis effiacy of plasma Exchange. *Intern. Med. J.* 2012; 42: 95-8.

[127] Chen M-H, Chen M-H, Chen W-S, Chang PM-H, Lee H-T, Lin H-Y et al. Thrombotic microangiopathy in systemic lupus erythematosus: a cohort study in North Taiwan. *Rheumathology* 2011; 50: 768-75.

[128] Claridge S, Das P, Dorling A, Robson M. Plasmapheresis as rescue therapy for systemic lupus erthyematosus-associated diffuse alveolar haemorrhage. *BMJ Case Reports* 2011; doi: 10.1136/bcr.02.2011.3893

[129] Lumlertgul D, Suteeka Y, Tumpong S, Bunnachak D, Boonkaew. Double filtration plasmapheresis in different diseases in Thailand. *Therapeutic Apheresis and Dyalisis* 2013; 17 (1): 99-116.

[130] Fantò M, Salemi S, Socciarelli F, Bartolazzi A, Natale GA, Casorelli I, Pavan A, Vaglio S, Di Rosa R, D'Amelio R. A case report of subacute cutaneous lupus erythematosus in a patient with mixed connetive tissue

disease: Successful treatment with plasmapheresis and rituximab. *Case reports in Rheumathology*. Volume 2013, Article ID 857694.
[131] Stojan G, Baer AN, et al. Flares of systemic lupus erythematosus during pregnancy and the puerperium: prevention, diagnosis and management. *Expert Rev. Clin. Immunol.* 8(5), 439-453 (2012).
[132] Martin JN Jr, Bailey AP, Rehberg JF, Owens MT, Keiser SD, May WL. Thrombotic thrombocytopenic purpura in 166 pregnancies: 1955-2006. *Am. J. Obstet. Gynecol.* 199(2), 98–104 (2008).
[133] Ambros-Rudolph CM. Dermatoses of pregnancy-clues to diagnosis, fetal risk and therapy. *Ann. Dermatol.* 2011;23:265-75.
[134] Doblas PA, Eguiluz I, Barber MA, Hijano JV, Alonso L, López-Torres E, et al. Trastornos dermatológicos y gestación. *Clin. Invest. Gin. Obst.* 2002;29:254-60.
[135] Doblas PA, Barber MA, Eguiluz I, Andérica JR, Hijazo JV, Suárez M, et al. Herpes gestationis (penfigoide gestacional). *Clin. Invest. Gin. Obst.* 2004;31:62--6.
[136] Beard MP, Millington GWM. Recent developments in the specific dermatoses of pregnancy. *Clin. Exp. Dermatol.* 2011;37:1--5.
[137] Shimanovich I, Skrobek C, Rose C, et al. Pemphigoid gestationis with predominant involvement of oral mucous membranes and IgA autoantibodies targeting the C-terminus of BP180. *J. Am. Acad. Dermatol.* 2002; 47:780.
[138] Katz SI. Herpes gestationis (pemphigoid gestationis). In: Fitzpatrick's Dermatology in General Medicine, 5th ed, Freedberg I, Eisen AZ, Wolff K. et al. (Eds), McGraw-Hill, 1999. p.686.
[139] Jenkins RE, Hern S, Black MM. Clinical features and management of 87 patients with pemphigoid gestationis. *Clin. Exp. Dermatol.* 1999; 24:255.
[140] Roger D, Vaillant L, Fignon A, Pierre F, Bacq Y, Brechot JF, et al. Specific pruritic diseases of pregnancy. A prospective study of 3192 pregnant women. *Arch. Dermatol.* 1994;130:73-49.
[141] Holmes RC, Black MM. The specific dermatoses of pregnancy. *J. Am. Acad. Dermatol.* 1983;8:405--12.
[142] Borrego L, Iglesias L. Dermatosis específicas del embarazo. Actualización. *Actas Dermatosifiliogr.* 2002;93:159-67.
[143] Shoronick JK, Black MM. Fetal risk in herpes gestationis. *J. Am. Acad. Dermatol.* 1992;26:63-8.
[144] Uceda ME, Guillén M. Dermatoses in pregnancy. Presentation of a case. *Semergen.* 2014;40(1):e8-e13.

[145] Amato L, Mei S, Gallerani I, et al. A case of herpes gestationis: persistent disease or conversion to bullous pemphigoid. *J. Am. Acad. Dermatol.* 2003;49:302–7.
[146] Marker M, Derfler K, Monshi B, et al. Successful immunoapheresis of bullous autoimmune disease: pemphigus vulgaris and pemphigoid gestationis. *J. Dtsch. Dermatol. Ges*. 2011;9:27–31.
[147] Van de Wiel A, Hart CH, Flinterman J, et al. Plasma exchange in herpes gestationis. *Br. Med. J*. 1980;281: 1041–2.
[148] Fortson MR, Freedman SN, Webster PD 3rd. Clinical assessment of hyperlipidemic pancreatitis. *Am. J. Gastroenterol*. 1995; 90:2134.
[149] Chang CC, Hsieh YY, Tsai HD, et al. Acute pancreatitis in pregnancy. Zhonghua Yi Xue Za Zhi (Taipei) 1998; 61:85.
[150] Berglund L, Brunzell JD, Goldberg AC, et al. Evaluation and treatment of hypertriglyceridemia: an Endocrine Society clinical practice guideline. *J. Clin. Endocrinol. Metab*. 2012; 97:2969.
[151] Navina S, Acharya C, DeLany JP, et al. Lipotoxicity causes multisystem organ failure and exacerbates acute pancreatitis in obesity. *Sci. Transl. Med.* 2011; 3:107ra110.
[152] Fredrickson DS. An international classification of hyperlipidemias and hyperlipoproteinemias. *Ann. Intern. Med*. 1971; 75:471.
[153] Havel RJ. Familial dysbetalipoproteinemia. New aspects of pathogenesis and diagnosis. *Med. Clin. North Am.* 1982; 66:441.
[154] Rivellese AA, De Natale C, Di Marino L, et al. Exogenous and endogenous postprandial lipid abnormalities in type 2 diabetic patients with optimal blood glucose control and optimal fasting triglyceride levels. *J. Clin. Endocrinol. Metab.* 2004; 89:2153.
[155] Nair S, Yadav D, Pitchumoni CS. Association of diabetic ketoacidosis and acute pancreatitis: observations in 100 consecutive episodes of DKA. *Am. J. Gastroenterol*. 2000; 95:2795.
[156] Toskes PP. Hyperlipidemic pancreatitis. *Gastroenterol. Clin. North Am.* 1990; 19:783.
[157] Goldenberg NM, Wang P, Glueck CJ. An observational study of severe hypertriglyceridemia, hypertriglyceridemic acute pancreatitis, and failure of triglyceride-lowering therapy when estrogens are given to women with and without familial hypertriglyceridemia. *Clin. Chim. Acta* 2003; 332:11.
[158] Alagozlu H, Cindoruk M, Unal S. Tamoxifen-induced severe hypertriglyceridaemia and acute pancreatitis. *Clin. Drug Investig*. 2006; 26:297.

[159] Kekki M, Nikkila EA. Plasma triglyceride turnover during use of oral contraceptives. *Metabolism* 1971;21:878–879.

[160] Fahraeus L, Larsson-Cohn U, Wallentin L. Plasma lipoproteins including high density lipoprotein fractions during normal pregnancy. *Obstet. Gynecol.* 1985;66:468–472.

[161] Desoye G, Schweditsch MO, Pfeiffer KP, Zechner R, Kostner GM. Correlation of hormones with lipid and lipoprotein levels during pregnancy and postpartum. *J. Clin. Endocrinol. Metab.* 1987;64:704-712.

[162] Herrera E, Lasuncion MA, Gomez-Coronado D, Aranda P, López-Luna P, Maier I. Role of lipoprotein lipase activity on lipoprotein metabolism and fate of circulating triglycerides in pregnancy. *Am. J. Obstet. Gynecol.* 1988;158:1575–1583.

[163] Tsuang W, Navaneethan U, Ruiz L, et al. Hypertriglyceridemic pancreatitis: presentation and management. *Am. J. Gastroenterol.* 2009; 104:984.

[164] Ujházy E, Onderová E, Horá ková M, Bencová E, Durisová M, Nosál R, Balonová T, Zeljenková D. Teratological study of the hypolipidaemic drugs etofylline clofibrate (VULM) and fenofibrate in swiss mice. *Pharmacol. Toxicol.* 1989;64:286–290.

[165] Achard JM, Westeel PF, Moriniere P, et al. Pancreatitis related to severe acute hypertriglyceridemia during pregnancy: treatment with lipoprotein apheresis. *Intensive Care Med.* 1991; 17:236.

[166] Yamauchi H, Sunamura M, Takeda K, et al. Hyperlipidemia and pregnancy associated pancreatitis with reference to plasma exchange as a therapeutic intervention. *Tohoku J. Exp. Med.* 1986; 148:197.

[167] Gürsoy A, Kulaksizoglu M, Sahin M, et al. Severe hypertriglyceridemia-induced pancreatitis during pregnancy. *J. Natl. Med. Assoc.* 2006; 98:655.

[168] Sleth JC, Lafforgue E, Servais R, et al. [A case of hypertriglycideremia-induced pancreatitis in pregnancy: value of heparin]. *Ann. Fr. Anesth. Reanim.* 2004; 23:835.

[169] Furuya T, Komatsu M, Takahashi K, et al. Plasma exchange for hypertriglyceridemic acute necrotizing pancreatitis: report of two cases. *Ther. Apher.* 2002; 6:454.

[170] Stefanutti C, Di Giacomo S, Labbadia G. Timing clinical events in the treatment of pancreatitis and hypertriglyceridemia with therapeutic plasmapheresis. *Transfus. Apher. Sci.* 2011; 45:3.

[171] Yeh JH, Lee MF, Chiu HC. Plasmapheresis for severe lipemia: comparison of serum-lipid clearance rates for the plasma-exchange and double-filtration variants. *J. Clin. Apher.* 2003; 18:32.

[172] Praveen Sivakumaran, Steven W. Tabak, Kimberly Gregory, Samuel H. Pepkowitz, Ellen B. Klapper. Management of Familial Hypertriglyceridemia During Pregnancy With Plasma Exchange. Case report. *J. Clin. Apheresis* 2009; 24:42-46.

[173] Eckel RH. Lipoprotein lipase. A multifunctional enzyme relevant to common metabolic diseases. *N. Engl. J. Med.* 1989; 320:1060.

[174] Mikhail N, Trivedi K, Page C, et al. Treatment of severe hypertriglyceridemia in nondiabetic patients with insulin. *Am. J. Emerg. Med.* 2005; 23:415.

[175] KORN ED. Clearing factor, a heparin-activated lipoprotein lipase. I. Isolation and characterization of the enzyme from normal rat heart. *J. Biol. Chem.* 1955; 215:1.

[176] Loo CC, Tan JY. Decreasing the plasma triglyceride level in hypertriglyceridemia-induced pancreatitis in pregnancy: a case report. *Am. J. Obstet. Gynecol.* 2002; 187:241.

[177] Weintraub M, Rassin T, Eisenberg S, et al. Continuous intravenous heparin administration in humans causes a decrease in serum lipolytic activity and accumulation of chylomicrons in circulation. *J. Lipid Res.* 1994; 35:229.

[178] Sheehan H. The pathology of acute yellow atrophy and delayed chloroform poisoning. *J. Obstet. Gynaecol.* 1940; 47:49.

[179] Bacq Y, Riely CA. Acute fatty liver of pregnancy: the hepatologist's view. *Gastroenterologist* 1993; 1:257.

[180] Knight M, Nelson-Piercy C, Kurinczuk JJ, et al. A prospective national study of acute fatty liver of pregnancy in the UK. *Gut* 2008; 57:951.

[181] Castro MA, Fassett MJ, Reynolds TB, et al. Reversible peripartum liver failure: a new perspective on the diagnosis, treatment, and cause of acute fatty liver of pregnancy, based on 28 consecutive cases. *Am. J. Obstet. Gynecol.* 1999; 181:389.

[182] Ibdah JA. Acute fatty liver of pregnancy: an update on pathogenesis and clinical implications. *World J. Gastroenterol.* 2006;14;12(46):7397-404.

[183] Riely CA. Acute fatty liver of pregnancy. *Semin. Liver Dis.* 1987; 7:47.

[184] Wilcken B, Leung KC, Hammond J, et al. Pregnancy and fetal long-chain 3-hydroxyacyl coenzyme A dehydrogenase deficiency. *Lancet* 1993; 341:407.

[185] Treem WR, Rinaldo P, Hale DE, et al. Acute fatty liver of pregnancy and long-chain 3-hydroxyacyl-coenzyme A dehydrogenase deficiency. *Hepatology* 1994; 19:339.
[186] Sims HF, Brackett JC, Powell CK, et al. The molecular basis of pediatric long chain 3-hydroxyacyl-CoA dehydrogenase deficiency associated with maternal acute fatty liver of pregnancy. *Proc. Natl. Acad. Sci. U. S. A.* 1995; 92:841.
[187] Yang Z, Zhao Y, Bennett MJ, et al. Fetal genotypes and pregnancy outcomes in 35 families with mitochondrial trifunctional protein mutations. *Am. J. Obstet. Gynecol.* 2002; 187:715.
[188] Mansouri A, Fromenty B, Durand R, et al. Assessment of the prevalence of genetic metabolic defects in acute fatty liver of pregnancy (letter). *J. Hepatol.* (Denmark) 1996; 25:781.
[189] Bacq Y, Assor P, Gendrot C, et al. [Recurrent acute fatty liver of pregnancy]. *Gastroenterol. Clin. Biol.* 2007; 31:1135.
[190] Ibdah JA, Yang Z, Bennett MJ. Liver disease in pregnancy and fetal fatty acid oxidation defects. *Mol. Genet. Metab.* 2000;71:182-9.
[191] Matern D, Hart P, Murtha AP, et al. Acute fatty liver of pregnancy associated with short-chain acyl-coenzyme A dehydrogenase deficiency. *J. Pediatr.* 2001; 138:585.
[192] Bernuau J, Degott C, Nouel O, Rueff B, Benhamou JP. Non-fatal acute fatty liver of pregnancy. *Gut.* 1983 Apr;24(4):340-4.
[193] Castro MA, Ouzounian JG, Colletti PM, et al. Radiologic studies in acute fatty liver of pregnancy. A review of the literature and 19 new cases. *J. Reprod. Med.* 1996; 41:839.
[194] Ch'ng CL, Morgan M, Hainsworth I, Kingham JGC. Prospective study of liver dysfunction in pregnancy in Southwest Wales. *Gut.* 2002; 51(6):876–880.
[195] Bacq Y. Acute fatty liver of pregnancy. *Semin. Perinatol.* 1998; 22:134.
[196] Tang W, Huang Z, Wang Y, Bo H, Fu P. Effect of plasma exchange on hepatocyte oxidative stress, mitochondria function, and apoptosis in patients with acute fatty liver of pregnancy. *Artificial Organs.* 2012; 36(3):E39–E47.
[197] Mohammad Reza Seyyed Majidi, Jamshid Vafaeimanesh. Plasmapheresis in Acute Fatty Liver of Pregnancy: An Effective Treatment. *Case Rep. Obstet. Gynecol.* 2013; 2013: 615975.
[198] Jin F, Cao M, Bai Y, Zhang Y, Yang Y, Zhang B. Therapeutic effects of plasma exchange for the treatment of 39 patients with acute fatty liver of pregnancy. *Discovery Medicine.* 2012;13(72):369–373.

[199] Nelson DB, Yost NP, Cunningham FG. Acute fatty liver of pregnancy: clinical outcomes and expected duration of recovery. *Am. J. Obstet. Gynecol.* 2013; 209:456.e1.

In: Plasmapheresis and Intravenous … ISBN: 978-1-63117-916-7
Editor: Rossana Allegro

Chapter 4

EFFECTS OF IVIG ON T CELL FUNCTIONS

Lauriane Padet[1,2] and Renée Bazin[1,2,*]

[1]Department of Research and Development,
Héma-Québec, Québec, Canada
[2]Department of Biochemistry, Microbiology and
Bioinformatics, Laval University, Québec, Canada

ABSTRACT

Dysregulation of T cell functions results in the development and maintenance of autoimmune and systemic inflammatory disorders. In this context, CD4+ (helper) and CD8+ (cytotoxic) T cell activation leads to autoantibody production and self-reactive cytotoxicity respectively. IVIg is commonly used as a second line immunosuppressive therapy in patients suffering from these disorders. Over the past decades, clinical observations in IVIg-treated patients revealed significant modulations in T cell populations and functions (Th1/Th2 ratio, Treg numbers, cytokine expression, etc.). Similar observations on the immunomodulatory effects of IVIg on T cell populations (eg. activation and differentiation of various CD4+ subsets, reduction of CD8+ T cell cytotoxicity) were made using in vitro assays and animal models, suggesting that these experimental systems could be useful to decipher the mechanisms by which IVIg produces therapeutic effects in autoimmune and inflammatory disorders.

* Corresponding author: Renée Bazin, PhD. Department of R and D, Héma-Québec, 1070 Avenue des Sciences-de-la-Vie, Québec (Qc), Canada, G1V 5C3. Phone: (418) 780-4362, Fax: (418) 780-2091. E-mail: renee.bazin@hema-quebec.qc.ca.

In this chapter, we will review the various effects of IVIg on T cells both in vitro and in vivo. We will also summarize the mechanisms proposed to explain these effects and discuss the reasons for the discrepancies between conclusions drawn from studies published during the last decades.

INTRODUCTION

IVIg and Autoimmunity

IVIg has been used for several decades to treat an increasing number of autoimmune and inflammatory disorders. Excellent review articles on the clinical use of IVIg have been recently published and therefore, this issue will not be discussed in this chapter [1-7]. We will rather focus on the effects of IVIg in autoimmune diseases with an emphasis on T cells on the following sections, using clinical observations obtained from IVIg-treated patients and experimental data derived from in vitro work or in vivo experimentations using animal models of disease aimed at understanding the mechanisms of IVIg action. Indeed, it has been reported more than 30 years ago that modulations in T cell populations and functions were induced in IVIg-treated patients suffering from autoimmune disorders. For example, Th0 and Th2 anti-inflammatory responses have been documented in IVIg-treated patients [8-10].

Other studies have shown that the ratio of CD4+ T cell subpopulations (Th1/Th2) is decreased following IVIg treatment [11-15], consistent with the induction of immunosuppressive effects. In addition, these clinical observations have stimulated considerable research efforts to better understand the mechanisms by which the infusion of high dose IVIg results in modulations in lymphocyte populations and therapeutic effects in a variety of autoimmune and inflammatory disorders.

ROLE OF T CELLS IN AUTOIMMUNITY

T cells originate from lymphoid precursors in the bone marrow and migrate to the thymus where they differentiate. In the thymus, T cells reach a state in which they co-express the CD4 and CD8 molecules. These double positive cells are then first subjected to the process of positive selection, where a low affinity but sustained interaction between TCR and MHC molecules results in cell survival. Following positive selection, the expression of one of the two co-receptors CD4 and CD8 is lost. The negative selection process also occurs in the thymus, where dendritic cells and macrophages present self MHC/peptide complexes to CD4+ or CD8+ T cells. This selection process is essential to remove autoreactive T cells. High affinity interactions with the self MHC/peptide complexes result in apoptosis. At the end of the positive and negative selection processes, a repertoire of mature naive T cells competent against non self-antigens but tolerant to self-antigens is generated [16-19].

Naive T cells require 3 signals for activation which are provided by antigen presenting cells (APC) in the lymphoid organs [20-24]. The first signal consists in the recognition of MHC/peptide complexes by the TCR. CD8+ T cells interact specifically with MHC I/peptide complexes while CD4+ T cells interact with MHC II/peptide complexes. TCR engagement leads to interleukin (IL)-2 production, an important survival factor for T cells. However, TCR engagement is not sufficient for clonal expansion and T cell differentiation. A second signal is needed and provided following interaction between CD28 expressed on T cells and CD80/CD86 costimulatory molecules expressed on mature APC with the contribution of interactions between other pairs of costimulatory molecules. Such costimulatory signaling amplifies IL-2 production and increases the expression of the alpha chain of IL-2 receptor (CD25). The high affinity binding of IL-2 to its receptor induces T cell proliferation. In the absence of costimulatory signals, T cells cannot be fully activated and undergo apoptosis or become anergic [25-27]. The third signal required for T cell activation and differentiation into effector cell is provided by cytokines secreted by APC which upon binding to receptors on T cells provide signals critical for the determination of the appropriate type of immune response [22, 28].

Even though the machinery responsible to establish T cell tolerance to self-antigens is highly efficient, tolerance can be broken. Several contributing factors have been identified and include genetic predispositions, microbial infections or other environmental factors [29-34]. Cytotoxic T lymphocyte-associated antigen 4 (CTLA-4) [35], lymphoid protein tyrosine phosphate non-receptor type 22 (PTPN22) [36], T cell immunoglobulin and mucin-domain containing (TIM) family [37], autoimmune regulator gene (AIRE) [38] are examples of genes that can contribute to the development of autoimmunity. Some MHC alleles can induce over-expression of self-peptides and increase the likelihood of developing autoimmune diseases [39, 40]. Ineffective presentation of self-antigens in the thymus can also lead to autoimmunity by allowing survival of autoreactive T cells.

Microbial infections can trigger autoimmunity by creating a strong pro-inflammatory environment that can trigger nonspecific polyclonal activation of autoreactive T cells [31]. In addition, pathogens can induce autoreactive T cell activation by molecular mimicry or by causing damage to cells or tissues, leading to enhanced presentation of self-antigens. Finally, other environmental factors such as diet, drugs and pollution have been proposed as contributors to the development of autoimmunity [41-43]. In addition to activated autoreactive T cells, pathogenic autoantibodies are major contributors to the development of autoimmune disorders such as immune thrombocytopenia, type I diabetes, rheumatoid arthritis and multiple sclerosis [44-47]. In fact, the production of such antibodies by autoreactive B cells is highly dependent on autoreactive CD4+ helper T cells. Cytotoxic auto-reactive CD8+ T cells also play a predominant role in several autoimmune disorders such as type I diabetes [48], multiple sclerosis [49, 50], chronic inflammatory demyelinating polyneuropathy [51], stiff-person syndrome [52] and polymyositis [53] by mediating organ or tissue destruction. Autoreactive CD8+ T cells may also participate in the etiology of immune thrombocyto-penia [54]. Clearly, the different T cell subpopulations play a central role in the development of autoimmunity. Therefore, the clinical responses observed in many patients suffering from autoimmune disorders following IVIg administration have rapidly translated into the identification of T cells as potential direct or indirect targets of IVIg, given their major role in the pathophysiology of these diseases.

Is the Effect of IVIg on T Cells Direct or Indirect?: The Search for an Answer

A number of studies aimed at elucidating the mechanisms by which IVIg can affect T cell functions have been reported in the literature.

These studies were done either in ex vivo experimental systems or using animal models of disease. A summary of these investigations is presented in the following paragraphs.

Studies on Mitogen-Activated T Cells

In the 90s, several research groups have focused on the effect of IVIg on the functions of activated T cells using mitogen stimulation to mimic T cell activity during autoimmune disease. Phorbol esters such as phorbol myristate acetate (PMA) and phorbol dibutyrate (PDB) in combination with calcium ionophores (ionomycin) bypass surface TCR engagement and cross-linking requirements to directly activate intracellular signaling pathways leading to T cell activation [55, 56].

Using this experimental approach, opposing conclusions have been reached by different research groups. Some studies showed that IVIg decreased T cell activation upon peripheral blood mononuclear cell (PBMC) stimulation with PMA/ionomycin. More precisely, IVIg reduced the secretion of cytokines such as IL-2, IFN-γ, TNF-β and others, as well as T cell proliferation as evaluated by [^{3}H]thymidine incorporation [57, 58].

A similar study performed on purified T cells activated with PMA/ionomycin rather than PBMC also described the IVIg-mediated inhibition of IL-2 secretion, suggesting that IVIg exerts its anti-inflammatory effect by acting directly on T cells [59]. This inhibitory effect was not the consequence of cell death or repression of IL-2 mRNA expression [57, 59]. Therefore, a post-transcriptional regulation of IL-2 by IVIg was proposed to explain the inhibition of IL-2 secretion but the precise mechanisms by which IVIg affected T cell activation remained unclear [59].

Interestingly, another group reached an opposing conclusion following the demonstration of the absence of inhibitory effect of IVIg on T cells after PBMC or purified T cell stimulation with PDB/ionomycin [60].

The reason for this discrepancy is unclear since phorbol esters such as PMA and PDB produce similar effects on T cells. Another study provided new insights into the inhibitory mechanisms of IVIg by showing that IVIg inhibited T cell activation by PMA/ionomycin, but only when PBMC and not purified T cells were used [58].

These latter results suggested that accessory cells (B cells, monocytes) from PBMC were required for IVIg to exert its anti-inflammatory effect on T cells and support an indirect rather than direct effect of IVIg on T cells. It has also been suggested that IVIg modulated T cell functions by inducing soluble anti-inflammatory factors such as IL-1RA [61]. IL-1RA competes with IL-1 for the binding to the IL-1 receptor and thus deprives T cells of important activation signals [62].

In summary, although interesting data have emerged from studies using T cells activated with phorbol esters and ionomycin, the results obtained by various groups of investigators did not permit to clarify the exact mechanism by which IVIg affects T cell populations in IVIg-treated patients.

Studies on Lectin-Activated T Cells

Lectins such as phytohemagglutinin (PHA), concanavalin A (ConA) and pokeweed mitogen (PWM) have also been used to study the effect of IVIg on T cell functions [63-72]. Lectins are sugar-binding proteins able to bind cell surface carbohydrates on T cells, leading to their aggregation and subsequent activation [73]. Several studies showed that IVIg inhibited T cell proliferation, CD25 expression and IFN-γ secretion upon PBMC stimulation with PHA [64, 70, 72]. Similar results were obtained with purified T cells or T cell lines stimulated with PHA, suggesting that IVIg directly affected the functions of activated T cells [59, 69]. The inhibitory effect of IVIg on T cell was reported to be partially due to apoptosis induction [70], in contradiction with the results obtained with T cells activated with phorbol esters/ionomycin discussed above, in which T cell viability was not affected by IVIg [57, 59].

Overall, studies with T cells activated with phorbol esters/ionomycin and lectins did not permit to reach a consensus as to whether IVIg effects are a consequence of a direct or indirect action on these cells.

Recent data from our laboratory permitted to revisit the different conclusions from previous works using mitogen-activated T cells. Indeed, we showed that the putative inhibitory effect of IVIg on activated T cell functions was in fact the consequence of lectin neutralization by IVIg [74]. Lectins such as PHA are able to bind to immunoglobulins through the recognition of biantennary oligosaccharides found on the Fab region of some IgG [75-77].

Therefore, the experimental design used in the study of the effects of IVIg on lectin-stimulated T cells should have taken into account the possibility of mitogen neutralization, especially when IVIg is present at the same time as the lectin, which was the case in most of the above-mentioned studies. In our studies, we depleted IVIg preparations of PHA-reactive IgG and showed the absence of inhibitory effect of these depleted IVIg preparations when added together with PHA to T cell cultures. These results clearly demonstrated that the previously reported inhibitory effect of IVIg on lectin-activated T cells was the consequence of lectin neutralization rather than a direct effect of IVIg on T cells.

Studies on CD3/CD28-Activated T Cells

In addition to studies in which T cells were activated with mitogens or lectins, a number of studies have been performed with T cells stimulated with monoclonal anti-CD3 antibodies to induce T cell activation in a more physiologically relevant manner [78]. In these studies, anti-CD3 addition to PBMC cultures resulted in T cell proliferation. However, in the presence of IVIg, the functions of anti-CD3 activated T cells were reported to be significantly decreased [57, 58, 60]. Interestingly, it was shown that anti-CD3 activated T cells were affected by IVIg when accessory cells were present in the cultures. In contrast, addition of IVIg to purified T cells in the presence of anti-CD3 did not prevent T cell activation [58], suggesting that accessory cells (B cells and/or monocytes) were required for the inhibitory effect of IVIg. In fact, T cells need costimulatory signals provided by accessory cells (e.g., CD80) for optimal activation with anti-CD3 antibodies [79-82]. Binding of human IgG to FcγR was shown to reduce the expression of CD80 on monocytes [83], suggesting that IVIg inhibited the anti-CD3-mediated T cell activation by decreasing costimulatory signals delivered by accessory cells to T cells [58].

In the light of the above observations on the role of accessory cells, the conclusions derived from studies reporting inhibitory effects of IVIg on activated purified T cells [59, 60] should be revisited. In fact, several studies showed that highly purified T cells cannot be fully activated with PMA/ionomycin or anti-CD3 in the absence of accessory cells [79, 84].

Therefore, one might consider that the above-mentioned studies with purified T cells were in fact done in the presence of a small amount of accessory cells, allowing T cell activation in the control conditions and IVIg-mediated inhibition in the experimental conditions. In fact, the early methods used to purify T cells included E-rosetting and nylon wool columns which do not yield a degree of purity as high as the more recent methods using positive selection with magnetic beads. Nevertheless, highly purified T cells can be activated in the absence of accessory cells using a combination of anti-CD3 and anti-CD28 [85]. Using this strategy, a group of investigators reported a partial but significant inhibition of highly purified T cell proliferation in the presence of IVIg [67], once again raising the possibility of a direct effect of IVIg on T cells. However, this possibility has been challenged recently in a study from our laboratory showing that IVIg can neutralize CD3/CD28 T cell expander beads, which are microbeads coated with anti-CD3 and anti-CD28 antibodies that are known to be very potent T cell activators. In fact, IVIg interfered with the binding of anti-CD3/CD28-coated microbeads to the T cells, thereby preventing activation [86]. Control experiments showed that prior incubation of purified T cells with IVIg did not affect the ability of CD3/CD28 beads to activate T cells and that IVIg did not affect the functions of T cells pre-activated with anti-CD3/CD28 beads [86].

In summary, the results derived from all the aforementioned in vitro studies must be interpreted with caution. A lesson can be learned from all these studies: experimental systems should be tightly controlled to rule out bystander effects or other possible interferences before making definitive conclusions on the mechanisms of action of IVIg on T cells.

Studies on CD4+ T Cell Subpopulations

The Th1/Th2 Subsets

CD4+ T cells can differentiate into various subpopulations of effector cells including T-helper 1 (Th1) and Th2 designed to eliminate different types of pathogens. Th1 and Th2 responses are elicited by professional APC and are characterized by their cytokine secretion profile [87-89]. The hallmark of a Th1 response is the production of interferon-gamma (IFN-γ) which activates the bactericidal activity of macrophages and induces the production of opsonizing and complement-fixing antibodies by B cells. The Th1 response is therefore important for the induction of cell-mediated immunity and plays a crucial role in the defence against intracellular pathogens [90]. On the other hand, the Th2 response is characterized by the secretion of IL-4, IL-5 and IL-13 and induces the production of neutralizing non-cytolytic antibodies by B cells, leading to humoral immunity. Th2 responses play a critical role in the defence against extracellular bacteria, parasites including helminths and toxins [91].

Early studies have associated the development of autoimmunity with a shift towards Th1 responses while a shift towards Th2 responses was believed to alleviate the disease [92, 93]. More recently this Th1/Th2 paradigm has been revisited since Th2 responses have also been implicated in autoimmune diseases, highlighting the complexity of immune response in autoimmunity [94].

Still, the Th1/Th2 concept continues to be accepted as part of the complex interactions observed during the development of autoimmune diseases. Therefore, restoration of the Th1/Th2 balance has been proposed as a therapeutic approach for the treatment of autoimmune disorders [95, 96].

Interestingly, several clinical studies have shown that IVIg modulated the Th1/Th2 ratio in favour of Th2 responses [8-10].

In autoimmune disorders, CD4+ T cells are activated following presentation of autoantigens by APC. Therefore, to study the mechanisms by which IVIg affects the CD4+ T cell response in a context relevant to autoimmunity, we first used a mouse model of immunization using ovalbumin (OVA) as an antigen and evaluated the impact of IVIg infusion during the immunization period on the generation of OVA-specific T cells [97]. Using this strategy, we showed that IVIg significantly reduced the number of OVA-specific T cells produced in response of OVA immunization. We also showed that the in vivo activation of OVA-specific CD4+ T cells from transgenic mice expressing a rearranged TCR transgene specific for the I-Ad–$OVA_{323–339}$ complex [98] was reduced in the presence of IVIg. These results thus confirmed the effect of IVIg on antigen-specific CD4+ T cells, but did not permit to determine whether the effect of IVIg on these cells was direct or indirect. To address more directly this question, we used an in vitro OVA presentation assay and demonstrated that the presence of IVIg during the incubation of APC with OVA greatly affected the ability of APC to activate OVA-specific CD4+ T cells. In contrast, OVA-loaded APC were able to efficiently activate OVA-specific CD4+ T cells in the presence or absence of IVIg. These results thus suggested that the inhibitory effect of IVIg was dependent on APC and not directly on the CD4+ T cells. Two mechanisms possibly involved in the inhibitory effect of IVIg on antigen presentation by APC were proposed. First, IVIg can compete with immune complexes of antigen for binding to FcγR, therefore reducing antigen internalization inside the APC. Second, IVIg can compete intracellularly with the internalized antigen for loading on MHC II molecules, thereby decreasing the amount of MHC II-peptide complexes presented on the surface of APC [99].

In summary, the above studies have revealed that IVIg does not directly affect the functions of CD4+ T cells but acts mainly by decreasing the ability of APC to present antigens in an MHC II-restricted manner. In the context of an autoimmune disease, this effect of IVIg could result in a reduced presentation of self-antigens to autoreactive CD4+ T cells and could thus contribute to the restore the Th1/Th2 ratio in IVIg-treated patients.

The Th17 Subset

Besides the classical Th1 and Th2 subsets, naive CD4+ T cells can also differentiate into other subsets of effector cells such as Th9, Th17 and Th22 [100]. The Th17 subset recently attracted much interest owing to its involvement in the development of autoimmune and inflammatory disorders [101, 102]. Th17 cells are characterized by the secretion of IL-17A, IL-17F, IL-21 and IL-22 and by the expression of transcription factors distinct from Th1 and Th2. These pro-inflammatory cells play a major role in the immune response against extracellular bacteria and fungi [103-105].

In addition, memory Th17 cells are drivers of chronic inflammation and this property has been strongly associated with many human autoimmune and chronic inflammatory disorders, including psoriasis, Crohn's disease, rheumatoid arthritis, multiple sclerosis and uveitis [106-110].

The involvement of Th17 cells in autoimmune disorders has prompted an analysis of this cell population in IVIg-treated patients suffering from inflammatory myopathies. An imbalance ratio of Th1/Th17 was observed in these patients before IVIg treatment. In IVIg responders, the ratio of Th1/Th17 cells was lower than that observed in non-responders, suggesting a role for the Th17 mediated pathway in the anti-inflammatory response of IVIg [111]. The effect of IVIg on Th17 cells was also recently studied using a mouse model of EAE, an experimental model of multiple sclerosis [112].

In this model, the pathogenesis was improved by IVIg treatment and this effect was associated with a decreased number of Th17 cells in the draining lymph nodes and spleen. Based on their results in the mouse model of EAE, the authors proposed that the anti-inflammatory activity of IVIg could be mediated either by a direct interaction of IVIg with T cells or by modulating the functions of APCs. The same group of investigators also studied the effects of IVIg on Th17 cells in vitro, starting with CD4+ T cells stimulated with monoclonal anti-CD3 and anti-CD28 antibodies in the presence of selected cytokines [113]. They showed that IVIg prevented the differentiation of CD4+ T cells into Th17 cells [114] and proposed that this effect was related to the inhibition of phosphorylation of the signal transducer and activator of transcription 3 (Stat3), a transcription factor that plays a central role in the differentiation and stabilization of the Th17 lineage [115, 116]. It has been shown that CD3 ligation by monoclonal antibodies induces tyrosine and serine phosphorylation of Stat3 in human CD4+ T cells [117]. Considering that anti-CD3/CD28 stimulation was used to trigger the activation of CD4+ T cells prior to their differentiation into Th17 cells, a possible interference between IVIg and antibodies used for activation cannot be excluded to in part explain the inhibitory effect of IVIg on the differentiation of CD4+ T cells, as previously discussed [74, 86].

Therefore, the elucidation of a direct or indirect effect of IVIg on Th17 cells will require further investigation in clinical studies with IVIg-treated patients, in animal models of diseases with a known Th17 component and also using in vitro systems with well-controlled experimental conditions.

Regulatory T Cells

Regulatory T cells (Tregs) have been originally described by Shimon Sakaguchi [118, 119] and were later characterized as CD4+ CD25^{high} Foxp3+ T cells [120]. Most Tregs are formed during T cell maturation in the thymus, where some T cells specific for self-antigens are not eliminated through the process of negative selection but instead differentiate into natural Foxp3+ Tregs. These cells were initially named natural Tregs or nTregs and represent about 5 % of the total CD4+ T cells in circulation [121]. Recently, a panel of experts recommended that Tregs originating from the thymus should be named thymus-derived Tregs (tTregs) instead of nTregs [122].

tTregs are indispensable for the maintenance of homeostasis and peripheral tolerance and for the prevention of autoimmunity [123, 124]. In addition to tTregs, other Tregs have been described and arise from naive autoreactive T cells in the periphery under certain environmental conditions such as the composition of the cytokine milieu, the concentration of antigen and the nature of the antigen-presenting cells [125, 126]. The newly proposed nomenclature for these cells is peripherally-derived Treg (pTreg) instead of the previously used terms such as induced Tregs (iTregs) or adaptive Tregs (aTregs), and the word iTregs should now refer to in vitro-induced Tregs (iTregs) [122]. The importance of CD4+ CD25^{high} Foxp3+ Tregs in the control of autoimmunity has been revealed following the identification of loss-of-function mutations in the Foxp3 gene leading to the immunodysregulation polyendocrinopathy enteropathy X-linked (IPEX) syndrome [127-129].

Foxp3 is considered to be the master regulator of the Treg lineage. In the IPEX syndrome, the lack of Tregs is associated with a lethal auto-aggressive lymphoproliferation, highlighting the prime importance of Tregs for the prevention of autoimmunity.

Since that discovery, the development of a number of autoimmune diseases such as ITP [130, 131], SLE [132], Kawasaki disease [133], Guillain-Barré syndrome [134], type I diabetes [135, 136], multiple sclerosis [137, 138] has been associated with anomalies in Treg numbers or immunosuppressive functions.

Several clinical studies on IVIg-treated patients suffering from autoimmune disorders have revealed modulations in Treg populations.

For example, increased numbers of circulating Tregs have been reported in Kawasaki disease [133, 139], Guillain-Barré syndrome [134], eosinophilic granulomatosis [140] and autoimmune rheumatic disease [141] following IVIg infusion. The effect of IVIg on Tregs has also been studied in animal models of disease.

In the EAE mouse model, repeated injections of IVIg were shown to prevent the development of the disease. The protection was associated with increased numbers of tTregs in the blood, lymph nodes and spleen [142]. A further demonstration of the role of Tregs for the effects of IVIg in this model was the failure of IVIg to protect against EAE in mice that were depleted of Tregs. The effect of IVIg was also studied in a mouse model of herpes simplex virus-induced encephalitis, in which a single dose of IVIg was sufficient to increase the number of Tregs in peripheral lymphoid organs and protect mice against HSV infection.

The underlying mechanism for this effect was the induction by IVIg of a subset of IL-10-producing FoxP3- ICOS+ CD4+ T cells [143]. Another study revealed that IVIg ameliorated the OVA-induced airway hyperresponsiveness in mice by increasing pTreg numbers by a factor of 4 to 6 times [144].

In this latter model, the induction of OVA-specific pTregs was mediated by tolerogenic APC generated after IVIg exposure. This observation supports an indirect rather than direct effect of IVIg on this Treg population, in contrast with the observation done using the EAE model, in which a direct effect of IVIg on tTreg proliferation was reported [142].

In vitro studies have permitted to show a direct effect of IVIg on purified CD4+ tTregs from healthy individuals, leading to their activation and increased expression of CD69, CD38, HLA-DR, IL-10, TGF-β and FoxP3 [145, 146].

On the other hand, the generation of pTregs from naive T cells in the periphery seems to be rather an indirect consequence of the effect of IVIg on APC, leading to the generation of tolerogenic dendritic cells (DC) [144, 147, 148].

Recently, De Groot et al. described the occurrence of short sequences of amino acid (Tregitopes) present within the structure of the IgG molecule able to induce the expansion of CD4+ Tregs [149]. The corresponding peptides (also termed Tregitopes) were synthesized and shown to induce tTreg and pTreg (adaptive or antigen-specific Treg) activation and expansion following binding to MHC II molecules of APC, both in vitro and in vivo [149-151]. Since IVIg has been shown to be internalized inside APC [99, 152, 153], it can be speculated that Tregitopes derived from internalized IVIg are loaded onto MHC II molecules and presented by APC in IVIg-treated patients, therefore providing an additional explanation for the expansion and stimulation of Tregs following IVIg therapy [154, 155].

Studies on CD8+ T Cells

Many subpopulations of cytotoxic CD8+ T cells have been defined based on their cytokine secretion profile. Type 1 CD8+ T cells (Tc1) secrete IFN-γ, whereas Tc2 secrete IL-4 and IL-5. Tc17 secrete IL-17 whereas CD8+ Tregs act through the secretion of both TGF-β and IL-10 [156, 157]. Altogether, CD8+ T cells play a major role in immunity against viruses and cancer. These cells acquire their cytotoxic function upon recognition by their TCR of MHC I-peptide complexes expressed on target cells. Cytotoxic CD8+ T cells rapidly destroy target cells following release of lytic granules (perforin, granzyme) or by expressing factors capable of signaling through death receptors expressed on the surface of target cells (FAS pathway) [158-160]. However, dysregulation in CD8+ T cells tolerance to self-antigens directly contributes to the initiation, progression and regulation of several autoimmune diseases such as type I diabetes, multiple sclerosis and others [161].

Data from clinical studies with IVIg-treated patients have shown a reduction in CD8+ T cell numbers in Crohn's disease [162] as well as a normalization of the CD8+ T cell repertoire in CIDP patients following high-dose IVIg infusion [163]. To better understand the effect of IVIg on CD8+ T cells observed in these clinical studies, we used a mouse model of OVA immunization similar to that described for the work on CD4+ T cells in Aubin et al. [164]. IVIg was administered at different intervals during the immunization of C57/BL6 mice with OVA. In these experiments, the number of CD8+ OVA-specific T cells was significantly lower in IVIg-treated animals, as evaluated using SINNFEKL-specific MHC I tetramers, in agreement with the clinical data. To decipher the mechanisms of IVIg effect on the CD8+ T cell response, an in vitro activation system using antigen cross-presentation was set up, in which APC cross-presented OVA peptides to OVA-specific CD8+ T cells (OT-I) purified from the spleen of mice expressing a rearranged TCR transgene specific for the H2-Kb-OVA$_{257–264}$ complex [165]. This assay permitted to show that IVIg inhibited the activation of OVA-specific CD8+ T cells when the antigen was added in the form of an immune complex (OVA-IC) [166]. The mechanism responsible for this inhibition was similar to that observed for the inhibition of the CD4+ T cell response, namely a competition between IVIg and OVA-IC for the binding to FcγR expressed on APC, resulting in a decreased presentation of MHC I-peptide (SIINFEKL) complexes and consequently, a reduction in OVA-specific CD8+ T cell activation. Interestingly, an additional mechanism was revealed in experiments done with OVA-preloaded APC incubated with OVA-specific CD8+ T cells in the presence or absence of IVIg. In the presence of IVIg, a significant reduction in OVA-specific CD8+ T cell activation and proliferation was observed, in contrast to the absence of IVIg effect on CD4+ T cells using a similar experimental approach [99].

Given that the expression of key costimulatory molecules on APC can be reduced following IVIg treatment [167], we speculate that this reduction may have a more drastic consequence on CD8+ compared to CD4+ T cell activation. Alternatively, IVIg may act by preventing the interaction between costimulatory molecules important for CD8+ but not CD4+ T cell activation.

In parallel, experiments addressing the cytotoxic activity of OVA-specific CD8+ T cells on target cells were performed both in vivo and in vitro. OVA immunization of C57/BL6 mice in the presence of IVIg resulted in a decreased number of perforin- and CD107a (a cell surface marker associated with degranulation)-expressing CD8+ T cells in the spleen [164].

In addition, OVA-specific CD8+ T cells activated following cross-presentation of OVA were less cytotoxic for their target cells (EL-4 decorated with SIINFEKL peptides) when IVIg was present during the incubation between activated CD8+ T cells and EL-4 cells.

This latter effect was shown to be related to TCR blockade by IVIg, thereby reducing the interaction between effector and target cells [164].

Altogether, the results from our studies on CD8+ T cells revealed that the effect of IVIg on their activation is, at least in part, the consequence of antigen cross-presentation impairment. As discussed above, interference of IVIg with the antigen presentation process also prevents CD4+ T cell activation, supporting the concept of an indirect rather than direct effect of IVIg on T cells. Yet, our work on CD8+ T cells also revealed a direct effect of IVIg on CD8+ T cell activation that was not observed on CD4+ T cells. Similarly, we showed that IVIg directly affects CD8+ T cell cytotoxicity, possibly as a consequence of TCR blockade. These latter results suggest that direct effects of IVIg on T cells synergize with the effects on antigen presentation to produce immunosuppressive effects in treated patients.

Conclusion

Altogether, the studies using ex-vivo experimental systems or animal models of disease suggest that the inhibitory effect of IVIg on T cells is mostly the indirect consequence of an effect of IVIg on APC (decreased self-antigen presentation, generation of tolerogenic dendritic cells).

Nevertheless, several studies showed that IVIg selectively modulates the functions of T cell subpopulations (inhibition of Th17 differentiation, decrease cytotoxicity of activated CD8+ T cells, induction of Tregs with strong immunosuppressive potential). Overall, the studies done during the past decades on the effects of IVIg on T cells have revealed a diversity of mechanisms by which immunosuppression can occur. However, much work remains to be done to fully understand and control the effectiveness of IVIg therapy in a variety of autoimmune and inflammatory disorders.

ACKNOWLEDGMENTS

The authors wish to thank Dr. Lionel Loubaki for helpful advices and careful reading of the manuscript.

REFERENCES

[1] Berger, M. Subcutaneous IgG in neurologic diseases. *Immunotherapy* 2014,6:71-83.

[2] Cakmak, S. K., Cakmak, A., Gonul, M., A. Klc, Gul, U. Intravenous immunoglobulin therapy in dermatology: an update. *Inflamm. Allergy Drug Targets* 2013,12:132-146.

[3] Gelfand, E. W. Intravenous immune globulin in autoimmune and inflammatory diseases. *N. Engl. J. Med.* 2012,367:2015-2025.

[4] Imbach, P. 30 years of immunomodulation by intravenous immunoglobulin. *Immunotherapy* 2012,4:651-654.

[5] Imbach, P. Treatment of immune thrombocytopenia with intravenous immunoglobulin and insights for other diseases. A historical review. *Swiss Med. Wkly.* 2012,142:w13593.

[6] Navarro, R. P., Ballow, M., Fenrick, B., Pezalla, E. J. Considerations for the optimal use of immunoglobulin. *Am. J. Manag. Care* 2012,18:S67-78.

[7] Winkelmann, A., Zettl, U. K. Use of intravenous immunoglobulin in the treatment of immune-mediated demyelinating diseases of the nervous system. *Curr. Pharm. Des.* 2012,18:4570-4582.

[8] Graphou, O., Chioti, A., Pantazi, A., Tsukoura, C., Kontopoulou, V., Guorgiadou, E., et al. Effect of intravenous immunoglobulin treatment

on the Th1/Th2 balance in women with recurrent spontaneous abortions. *Am. J. Reprod. Immunol.* 2003,49:21-29.

[9] Mouzaki, A., Theodoropoulou, M., Gianakopoulos, I., Vlaha, V., Kyrtsonis, M. C., Maniatis, A. Expression patterns of Th1 and Th2 cytokine genes in childhood idiopathic thrombocytopenic purpura (ITP) at presentation and their modulation by intravenous immunoglobulin G (IVIg) treatment: their role in prognosis. *Blood* 2002,100:1774-1779.

[10] Yamada, H., Morikawa, M., Furuta, I., Kato, E. H., Shimada, S., Iwabuchi, K., et al. Intravenous immunoglobulin treatment in women with recurrent abortions: increased cytokine levels and reduced Th1/Th2 lymphocyte ratio in peripheral blood. *Am. J. Reprod. Immunol.* 2003,49: 84-89.

[11] Bordet, J. C., Follea, G., Carosella, E., Dechavanne, M. Intravenous high-dose IgG therapy induced alterations of spleen lymphocyte IgM secretion and T cell subsets in patients with idiopathic thrombocytopenic purpura. *Thromb. Res.* 1987,47:165-174.

[12] Dammacco, F., Iodice, G., Campobasso, N. Treatment of adult patients with idiopathic thrombocytopenic purpura with intravenous immunoglobulin: effects on circulating T cell subsets and PWM-induced antibody synthesis in vitro. *Br. J. Haematol.* 1986,62:125-135.

[13] Kwak-Kim, J., Lee, S. K., Gilman-Sachs, A. Elevated Th1/Th2 cell ratios in a pregnant woman with a history of RSA, secondary Sjogren's syndrome and rheumatoid arthritis complicated with one fetal demise of twin pregnancy. *Am. J. Reprod. Immunol.* 2007,58:325-329.

[14] Pogliani, E. M., Della Volpe, A., Casaroli, I., Maffe, P. F., Corneo, G. Lymphocyte subsets in patients with idiopathic thrombocytopenic purpura during high-dose gamma globulin therapy. *Allergol. Immunopathol. (Madr.)* 1991,19:113-116.

[15] Tsubakio, T., Kurata, Y., Katagiri, S., Kanakura, Y., Tamaki, T., Kuyama, J., et al. Alteration of T cell subsets and immunoglobulin synthesis in vitro during high dose gamma-globulin therapy in patients with idiopathic thrombocytopenic purpura. *Clin. Exp. Immunol.* 1983,53: 697-702.

[16] Klein, L., Hinterberger, M., Wirnsberger, G., Kyewski, B. Antigen presentation in the thymus for positive selection and central tolerance induction. *Nat. Rev. Immunol.* 2009,9:833-844.

[17] Morris, G. P., Allen, P. M. How the TCR balances sensitivity and specificity for the recognition of self and pathogens. *Nat. Immunol.* 2012,13:121-128.

[18] Mouchess, M. L., Anderson, M. Central tolerance induction. *Curr. Top Microbiol. Immunol.* 2014,373:69-86.

[19] Starr, T. K., Jameson, S. C., Hogquist, K. A. Positive and negative selection of T cells. *Annu. Rev. Immunol.* 2003,21:139-176.

[20] Boyman, O., Sprent, J. The role of interleukin-2 during homeostasis and activation of the immune system. *Nat. Rev. Immunol.* 2012,12:180-190.

[21] Brownlie, R. J., Zamoyska, R. T cell receptor signalling networks: branched, diversified and bounded. *Nat. Rev. Immunol.* 2013,13:257-269.

[22] Curtsinger, J. M., Mescher, M. F. Inflammatory cytokines as a third signal for T cell activation. *Curr. Opin. Immunol.* 2010,22:333-340.

[23] Hivroz, C., Chemin, K., Tourret, M., Bohineust, A. Crosstalk between T lymphocytes and dendritic cells. *Crit. Rev. Immunol.* 2012,32:139-155.

[24] Leitner, J., Grabmeier-Pfistershammer, K., Steinberger, P. Receptors and ligands implicated in human T cell costimulatory processes. *Immunol. Lett.* 2010,128:89-97.

[25] Appleman, L. J., Boussiotis, V. A. T cell anergy and costimulation. *Immunol. Rev.* 2003,192:161-180.

[26] Baumann, S., Krueger, A., Kirchhoff, S., Krammer, P. H. Regulation of T cell apoptosis during the immune response. *Curr. Mol. Med.* 2002,2: 257-272.

[27] Saibil, S. D., Deenick, E. K., Ohashi, P. S. The sound of silence: modulating anergy in T lymphocytes. *Curr. Opin. Immunol.* 2007,19: 658-664.

[28] Gutcher, I., Becher, B. APC-derived cytokines and T cell polarization in autoimmune inflammation. *J. Clin. Invest.* 2007,117:1119-1127.

[29] Atassi, M. Z., Casali, P. Molecular mechanisms of autoimmunity. *Autoimmunity* 2008,41:123-132.

[30] Bogdanos, D. P., Smyk, D. S., Invernizzi, P., Rigopoulou, E. I., Blank, M., Sakkas, L., et al. Tracing environmental markers of autoimmunity: introducing the infectome. *Immunol. Res.* 2013,56:220-240.

[31] Christen, U., von Herrath, M. G. Initiation of autoimmunity. *Curr. Opin. Immunol.* 2004,16:759-767.

[32] Rose, A. M., Bell, L. C. Epistasis and immunity: the role of genetic interactions in autoimmune diseases. *Immunology* 2012,137:131-138.

[33] Selmi, C., Lu, Q., Humble, M. C. Heritability versus the role of the environment in autoimmunity. *J. Autoimmun.* 2012,39:249-252.

[34] Tiniakou, E., Costenbader, K. H., Kriegel, M. A. Sex-specific environmental influences on the development of autoimmune diseases. *Clin. Immunol.* 2013,149:182-191.

[35] Romo-Tena, J., Gomez-Martin, D., Alcocer-Varela, J. CTLA-4 and autoimmunity: new insights into the dual regulator of tolerance. *Autoimmun. Rev.* 2013,12:1171-1176.

[36] Bottini, N., Peterson, E. J. Tyrosine Phosphatase PTPN22: Multifunctional Regulator of Immune Signaling, Development, and Disease. *Annu. Rev. Immunol.* 2013.

[37] Li, Z., Ju, Z., Frieri, M. The T-cell immunoglobulin and mucin domain (Tim) gene family in asthma, allergy, and autoimmunity. *Allergy Asthma Proc.* 2013,34:e21-26.

[38] Arstila, T. P., Jarva, H. Human APECED; a Sick Thymus Syndrome? *Front Immunol.* 2013,4:313.

[39] Trowsdale, J., Knight, J. C. Major histocompatibility complex genomics and human disease. *Annu. Rev. Genomics Hum. Genet.* 2013,14:301-323.

[40] Tsai, S., Santamaria, P. MHC Class II Polymorphisms, Autoreactive T-Cells, and Autoimmunity. *Front Immunol.* 2013,4:321.

[41] Dedeoglu, F. Drug-induced autoimmunity. *Curr. Opin. Rheumatol.* 2009,21:547-551.

[42] Farhat, S. C., Silva, C. A., Orione, M. A., Campos, L. M., Sallum, A. M., Braga, A. L. Air pollution in autoimmune rheumatic diseases: a review. *Autoimmun. Rev.* 2011,11:14-21.

[43] Manzel, A., Muller, D. N., Hafler, D. A., Erdman, S. E., Linker, R. A., Kleinewietfeld, M. Role of "Western diet" in inflammatory autoimmune diseases. *Curr. Allergy Asthma Rep.* 2014,14:404.

[44] Imboden, J. B. The immunopathogenesis of rheumatoid arthritis. *Annu. Rev. Pathol.* 2009,4:417-434.

[45] La Torre, D. Immunobiology of beta-cell destruction. *Adv. Exp. Med. Biol.* 2012,771:194-218.

[46] McMillan, R. The pathogenesis of chronic immune thrombocytopenic purpura. *Semin. Hematol.* 2007,44:S3-S11.

[47] Reindl, M., Di Pauli, F., Rostasy, K., Berger, T. The spectrum of MOG autoantibody-associated demyelinating diseases. *Nat. Rev. Neurol.* 2013, 9:455-461.

[48] Bulek, A. M., Cole, D. K., Skowera, A., Dolton, G., Gras, S., Madura, F., et al. Structural basis for the killing of human beta cells by CD8(+) T cells in type 1 diabetes. *Nat. Immunol.* 2012,13:283-289.

[49] Deckert, M., Sanchez-Ruiz, M., Brunn, A., Schluter, D. Role of CD8 T-cell-mediated autoimmune diseases of the central nervous system. *Crit. Rev. Immunol.* 2010,30:311-326.

[50] Friese, M. A., Fugger, L. Pathogenic CD8(+) T cells in multiple sclerosis. *Ann. Neurol.* 2009,66:132-141.

[51] Schneider-Hohendorf, T., Schwab, N., Uceyler, N., Gobel, K., Sommer, C., Wiendl, H. CD8+ T-cell immunity in chronic inflammatory demyelinating polyradiculoneuropathy. *Neurology* 2012,78:402-408.

[52] Poh, M. Q., Simon, N. G., Buckland, M. E., Salisbury, E., Watson, S. Evidence of T-cell mediated neuronal injury in stiff-person syndrome with anti-amphiphysin antibodies. *J. Neurol. Sci.* 2013.

[53] Takahashi, A., Takeda, I., Kanno, T., Nakahara, T., Odajima, H., Kasukawa, R. CD8-positive T cell-induced liver damage was found in a patient with polymyositis. *Intern. Med.* 2006,45:1059-1063.

[54] Kashiwagi, H., Tomiyama, Y. Pathophysiology and management of primary immune thrombocytopenia. *Int. J. Hematol.* 2013,98:24-33.

[55] Chopra, R. K., Nagel, J. E., Chrest, F. J., Boto, W. M., Pyle, R. S., Dorsey, B., et al. Regulation of interleukin 2 and interleukin 2 receptor gene expression in human T cells: I. Effect of Ca2+-ionophore on phorbol myristate acetate co-stimulated cells. *Clin. Exp. Immunol.* 1987, 69: 433-440.

[56] Zlotnik, A., Daine, B. Activation of IL 1-dependent and IL 1-independent T cell lines by calcium ionophore and phorbol ester. *J. Immunol.* 1986,136:1033-1037.

[57] Andersson, U. G., Bjork, L., Skansen-Saphir, U., Andersson, J. P. Down-regulation of cytokine production and interleukin-2 receptor expression by pooled human IgG. *Immunology* 1993,79:211-216.

[58] Skansen-Saphir, U., Andersson, J., Bjork, L., Ekberg, C., Fehniger, T. E., Henter, J. I., et al. Down-regulation of lymphokine synthesis by intravenous gammaglobulin is dependent upon accessory cells. *Scand. J. Immunol.* 1998,47:229-235.

[59] Modiano, J. F., Amran, D., Lack, G., Bradley, K., Ball, C., Domenico, J., et al. Posttranscriptional regulation of T-cell IL-2 production by human pooled immunoglobin. *Clin. Immunol. Immunopathol.* 1997,83: 77-85.

[60] Amran, D., Renz, H., Lack, G., Bradley, K., Gelfand, E. W. Suppression of cytokine-dependent human T-cell proliferation by intravenous immunoglobulin. *Clin. Immunol. Immunopathol.* 1994,73:180-186.

[61] Arend, W. P., Leung, D. Y. IgG induction of IL-1 receptor antagonist production by human monocytes. *Immunol. Rev.* 1994,139:71-78.

[62] Arend, W. P., Welgus, H. G., Thompson, R. C., Eisenberg, S. P. Biological properties of recombinant human monocyte-derived interleukin 1 receptor antagonist. *J. Clin. Invest.* 1990,85:1694-1697.

[63] Heidt, S., Roelen, D. L., Eijsink, C., Eikmans, M., Claas, F. H., Mulder, A. Intravenous immunoglobulin preparations have no direct effect on B cell proliferation and immunoglobulin production. *Clin. Exp. Immunol.* 2009,158:99-105.

[64] Kawada, K., Terasaki, P. I. Evidence for immunosuppression by high-dose gammaglobulin. *Exp. Hematol.* 1987,15:133-136.

[65] Klaesson, S., Ringden, O., Markling, L., Remberger, M., Lundkvist, I. Immune modulatory effects of immunoglobulins on cell-mediated immune responses in vitro. *Scand. J. Immunol.* 1993,38:477-484.

[66] Kondo, N., Ozawa, T., Mushiake, K., Motoyoshi, F., Kameyama, T., Kasahara, K., et al. Suppression of immunoglobulin production of lymphocytes by intravenous immunoglobulin. *J. Clin. Immunol.* 1991, 11:152-158.

[67] MacMillan, H. F., Lee, T., Issekutz, A. C. Intravenous immunoglobulin G-mediated inhibition of T-cell proliferation reflects an endogenous mechanism by which IgG modulates T-cell activation. *Clin. Immunol.* 2009,132:222-233.

[68] Stohl, W. Modulation of the immune response by immunoglobulin for intravenous use. I. Inhibition of pokeweed mitogen-induced B cell differentiation. *Clin. Exp. Immunol.* 1985,62:200-207.

[69] Tawfik, D. S., Cowan, K. R., Walsh, A. M., Hamilton, W. S., Goldman, F. D. Exogenous immunoglobulin downregulates T-cell receptor signaling and cytokine production. *Pediatr. Allergy Immunol.* 2012,23: 88-95.

[70] Tha-In, T., Metselaar, H. J., Tilanus, H. W., Boor, P. P., Mancham, S., Kuipers, E. J., et al. Superior immunomodulatory effects of intravenous immunoglobulins on human T-cells and dendritic cells: comparison to calcineurin inhibitors. *Transplantation* 2006,81:1725-1734.

[71] Toyoda, M., Zhang, X., Petrosian, A., Galera, O. A., Wang, S. J., Jordan, S. C. Modulation of immunoglobulin production and cytokine mRNA expression in peripheral blood mononuclear cells by intravenous immunoglobulin. *J. Clin. Immunol.* 1994,14:178-189.

[72] Van Schaik, I. N., Lundkvist, I., Vermeulen, M., Brand, A. Polyvalent immunoglobulin for intravenous use interferes with cell proliferation in vitro. *J. Clin. Immunol.* 1992,12:325-334.

[73] Kay, J. E. Mechanisms of T lymphocyte activation. *Immunol. Lett.* 1991, 29:51-54.

[74] Padet, L., St-Amour, I., Aubin, E., Bazin, R. Neutralization of mitogenic lectins by intravenous immunoglobulin (IVIg) prevents T cell activation: does IVIg really have a direct effect on T cells? *Clin. Exp. Immunol.* 2011,166:352-360.

[75] Green, E. D., Baenziger, J. U. Oligosaccharide specificities of Phaseolus vulgaris leukoagglutinating and erythroagglutinating phytohemagglutinins. Interactions with N-glycanase-released oligosaccharides. *J. Biol. Chem.* 1987,262:12018-12029.

[76] Holland, M., Yagi, H., Takahashi, N., Kato, K., Savage, C. O., Goodall, D. M., et al. Differential glycosylation of polyclonal IgG, IgG-Fc and IgG-Fab isolated from the sera of patients with ANCA-associated systemic vasculitis. *Biochim. Biophys. Acta* 2006,1760:669-677.

[77] Jefferis, R. Glycosylation of recombinant antibody therapeutics. *Biotechnol. Prog.* 2005,21:11-16.

[78] Dixon, J. F., Law, J. L., Favero, J. J. Activation of human T lymphocytes by crosslinking of anti-CD3 monoclonal antibodies. *J. Leukoc. Biol.* 1989,46:214-220.

[79] Davis, L., Lipsky, P. E. Signals involved in T cell activation. II. Distinct roles of intact accessory cells, phorbol esters, and interleukin 1 in activation and cell cycle progression of resting T lymphocytes. *J. Immunol.* 1986,136:3588-3596.

[80] Umetsu, D. T., Katzen, D., Chatila, T., Miller, R., Jabara, H. H., Maher, M., et al. Requirements for activation of human peripheral blood T cells by mouse monoclonal antibodies to CD3. *Clin. Immunol. Immunopathol.* 1987,43:48-64.

[81] Verwilghen, J., Baroja, M. L., Van Vaeck, F., Van Damme, J., Ceuppens, J. L. Differences in the stimulating capacity of immobilized anti-CD3 monoclonal antibodies: variable dependence on interleukin-1 as a helper signal for T-cell activation. *Immunology* 1991,72:269-276.

[82] Williams, J. M., Deloria, D., Hansen, J. A., Dinarello, C. A., Loertscher, R., Shapiro, H. M., et al. The events of primary T cell activation can be staged by use of Sepharose-bound anti-T3 (64.1) monoclonal antibody and purified interleukin 1. *J. Immunol.* 1985,135:2249-2255.

[83] Barcy, S., Wettendorff, M., Leo, O., Urbain, J., Kruger, M., Ceuppens, J. L., et al. FcR cross-linking on monocytes results in impaired T cell stimulatory capacity. *Int. Immunol.* 1995,7:179-189.

[84] Schwartz, R. H. A cell culture model for T lymphocyte clonal anergy. *Science* 1990,248:1349-1356.

[85] Trickett, A., Kwan, Y. L. T cell stimulation and expansion using anti-CD3/CD28 beads. *J. Immunol. Methods* 2003,275:251-255.

[86] Padet, L., Bazin, R. IVIg prevents the in vitro activation of T cells by neutralizing the T cell activators. *Immunol. Lett.* 2013,150:54-60.

[87] Luckheeram, R. V., Zhou, R., Verma, A. D., Xia, B. CD4(+)T cells: differentiation and functions. *Clin. Dev. Immunol.* 2012,2012:925135.

[88] Yamane, H., Paul, W. E. Early signaling events that underlie fate decisions of naive CD4(+) T cells toward distinct T-helper cell subsets. *Immunol. Rev.* 2013,252:12-23.

[89] Mosmann, T. R., Cherwinski, H., Bond, M. W., Giedlin, M. A., Coffman, R. L. Two types of murine helper T cell clone. I. Definition according to profiles of lymphokine activities and secreted proteins. *J. Immunol.* 1986,136:2348-2357.

[90] Cope, A., Le Friec, G., Cardone, J., Kemper, C. The Th1 life cycle: molecular control of IFN-gamma to IL-10 switching. *Trends Immunol.* 2011,32:278-286.

[91] Li, Z., Zhang, Y., Sun, B. Current understanding of Th2 cell differentiation and function. *Protein Cell* 2011,2:604-611.

[92] Lafaille, J. J. The role of helper T cell subsets in autoimmune diseases. *Cytokine Growth Factor Rev.* 1998,9:139-151.

[93] Liblau, R. S., Singer, S. M., McDevitt, H. O. Th1 and Th2 CD4+ T cells in the pathogenesis of organ-specific autoimmune diseases. *Immunol. Today* 1995,16:34-38.

[94] Crane, I. J., Forrester, J. V. Th1 and Th2 lymphocytes in autoimmune disease. *Crit. Rev. Immunol.* 2005,25:75-102.

[95] Adorini, L., Guery, J. C., Trembleau, S. Manipulation of the Th1/Th2 cell balance: an approach to treat human autoimmune diseases? *Auto-immunity* 1996,23:53-68.

[96] Kidd, P. Th1/Th2 balance: the hypothesis, its limitations, and implications for health and disease. *Altern. Med. Rev.* 2003,8:223-246.

[97] Aubin, E., Lemieux, R., Bazin, R. Indirect inhibition of in vivo and in vitro T-cell responses by intravenous immunoglobulins due to impaired antigen presentation. *Blood* 2010,115:1727-1734.

[98] Shimonkevitz, R., Colon, S., Kappler, J. W., Marrack, P., Grey, H. M. Antigen recognition by H-2-restricted T cells. II. A tryptic ovalbumin peptide that substitutes for processed antigen. *J. Immunol.* 1984,133: 2067-2074.

[99] Aubin, E., Proulx, D. P., Trepanier, P., Lemieux, R., Bazin, R. Prevention of T cell activation by interference of internalized intravenous immunoglobulin (IVIg) with MHC II-dependent native antigen presentation. *Clin. Immunol.* 2011,141:273-283.

[100] Liu, Z., Fan, H., Jiang, S. CD4(+) T-cell subsets in transplantation. *Immunol. Rev.* 2013,252:183-191.

[101] McGeachy, M. J. Th17 memory cells: live long and proliferate. *J. Leukoc. Biol.* 2013,94:921-926.

[102] Kurebayashi, Y., Nagai, S., Ikejiri, A., Koyasu, S. Recent advances in understanding the molecular mechanisms of the development and function of Th17 cells. *Genes Cells* 2013,18:247-265.

[103] Kaufmann, S. H., Kuchroo, V. K. Th17 cells. *Microbes Infect.* 2009,11: 579-583.

[104] Korn, T., Bettelli, E., Oukka, M., Kuchroo, V. K. IL-17 and Th17 Cells. *Annu. Rev. Immunol.* 2009,27:485-517.

[105] Miossec, P., Korn, T., Kuchroo, V. K. Interleukin-17 and type 17 helper T cells. *N. Engl. J. Med.* 2009,361:888-898.

[106] Annunziato, F., Cosmi, L., Liotta, F., Maggi, E., Romagnani, S. Type 17 T helper cells-origins, features and possible roles in rheumatic disease. *Nat. Rev. Rheumatol,* 2009,5:325-331.

[107] Larsen, J. M., Bonefeld, C. M., Poulsen, S. S., Geisler, C., Skov, L. IL-23 and T(H)17-mediated inflammation in human allergic contact dermatitis. *J. Allergy Clin. Immunol.* 2009,123:486-492.

[108] Louten, J., Boniface, K., de Waal Malefyt, R. Development and function of TH17 cells in health and disease. *J. Allergy Clin. Immunol.* 2009,123: 1004-1011.

[109] Maddur, M. S., Miossec, P., Kaveri, S. V., Bayry, J. Th17 cells: biology, pathogenesis of autoimmune and inflammatory diseases, and therapeutic strategies. *Am. J. Pathol.* 2012,181:8-18.

[110] Van Beelen, A. J., Teunissen, M. B., Kapsenberg, M. L., de Jong, E. C. Interleukin-17 in inflammatory skin disorders. *Curr. Opin. Allergy Clin. Immunol.* 2007,7:374-381.

[111] Tournadre, A., Porcherot, M., Cherin, P., Marie, I., Hachulla, E., Miossec, P. Th1 and Th17 balance in inflammatory myopathies: inter-

action with dendritic cells and possible link with response to high-dose immunoglobulins. *Cytokine* 2009,46:297-301.

[112] Othy, S., Hegde, P., Topcu, S., Sharma, M., Maddur, M. S., Lacroix-Desmazes, S., et al. Intravenous gammaglobulin inhibits encephalitogenic potential of pathogenic T cells and interferes with their trafficking to the central nervous system, implicating sphingosine-1 phosphate receptor 1-mammalian target of rapamycin axis. *J. Immunol.* 2013,190: 4535-4541.

[113] Maddur, M. S., Vani, J., Hegde, P., Lacroix-Desmazes, S., Kaveri, S. V., Bayry, J. Inhibition of differentiation, amplification, and function of human TH17 cells by intravenous immunoglobulin. *J. Allergy Clin. Immunol.* 2011,127:823-830 e821-827.

[114] Maddur, M. S., Kaveri, S. V., Bayry, J. Comparison of different IVIg preparations on IL-17 production by human Th17 cells. *Autoimmun. Rev.* 2011,10:809-810.

[115] Harris, T. J., Grosso, J. F., Yen, H. R., Xin, H., Kortylewski, M., Albesiano, E., et al. Cutting edge: An in vivo requirement for STAT3 signaling in TH17 development and TH17-dependent autoimmunity. *J. Immunol.* 2007,179:4313-4317.

[116] Ma, C. S., Chew, G. Y., Simpson, N., Priyadarshi, A., Wong, M., Grimbacher, B., et al. Deficiency of Th17 cells in hyper IgE syndrome due to mutations in STAT3. *J. Exp. Med.* 2008,205:1551-1557.

[117] Gerwien, J., Nielsen, M., Labuda, T., Nissen, M. H., Svejgaard, A., Geisler, C., et al. Cutting edge: TCR stimulation by antibody and bacterial superantigen induces Stat3 activation in human T cells. *J. Immunol.* 1999,163:1742-1745.

[118] Sakaguchi, S., Fukuma, K., Kuribayashi, K., Masuda, T. Organ-specific autoimmune diseases induced in mice by elimination of T cell subset. I. Evidence for the active participation of T cells in natural self-tolerance; deficit of a T cell subset as a possible cause of autoimmune disease. *J. Exp. Med.* 1985,161:72-87.

[119] Sakaguchi, S., Sakaguchi, N., Asano, M., Itoh, M., Toda, M. Immunologic self-tolerance maintained by activated T cells expressing IL-2 receptor alpha-chains (CD25). Breakdown of a single mechanism of self-tolerance causes various autoimmune diseases. *J. Immunol.* 1995, 155:1151-1164.

[120] Hori, S., Nomura, T., Sakaguchi, S. Control of regulatory T cell development by the transcription factor Foxp3. *Science* 2003,299:1057-1061.

[121] Allan, S. E., Alstad, A. N., Merindol, N., Crellin, N. K., Amendola, M., Bacchetta, R., et al. Generation of potent and stable human CD4+ T regulatory cells by activation-independent expression of FOXP3. *Mol. Ther.* 2008,16:194-202.
[122] Abbas, A. K., Benoist, C., Bluestone, J. A., Campbell, D. J., Ghosh, S., Hori, S., et al. Regulatory T cells: recommendations to simplify the nomenclature. *Nat. Immunol.* 2013,14:307-308.
[123] Ohkura, N., Kitagawa, Y., Sakaguchi, S. Development and maintenance of regulatory T cells. *Immunity* 2013,38:414-423.
[124] Wan, Y. Y. Regulatory T cells: immune suppression and beyond. *Cell Mol. Immunol.* 2010,7:204-210.
[125] Bluestone, J. A., Abbas, A. K. Natural versus adaptive regulatory T cells. *Nat. Rev. Immunol.* 2003,3:253-257.
[126] Lohr, J., Knoechel, B., Abbas, A. K. Regulatory T cells in the periphery. *Immunol. Rev.* 2006,212:149-162.
[127] Bennett, C. L., Christie, J., Ramsdell, F., Brunkow, M. E., Ferguson, P. J., Whitesell, L., et al. The immune dysregulation, polyendocrinopathy, enteropathy, X-linked syndrome (IPEX) is caused by mutations of FOXP3. *Nat. Genet.* 2001,27:20-21.
[128] Gambineri, E., Torgerson, T. R., Ochs, H. D. Immune dysregulation, polyendocrinopathy, enteropathy, and X-linked inheritance (IPEX), a syndrome of systemic autoimmunity caused by mutations of FOXP3, a critical regulator of T-cell homeostasis. *Curr. Opin. Rheumatol.* 2003, 15:430-435.
[129] Wildin, R. S., Ramsdell, F., Peake, J., Faravelli, F., Casanova, J. L., Buist, N., et al. X-linked neonatal diabetes mellitus, enteropathy and endocrinopathy syndrome is the human equivalent of mouse scurfy. *Nat. Genet.* 2001,27:18-20.
[130] Liu, B., Zhao, H., Poon, M. C., Han, Z., Gu, D., Xu, M., et al. Abnormality of CD4(+)CD25(+) regulatory T cells in idiopathic thrombocytopenic purpura. *Eur. J. Haematol.* 2007,78:139-143.
[131] Sakakura, M., Wada, H., Tawara, I., Nobori, T., Sugiyama, T., Sagawa, N., et al. Reduced Cd4+Cd25+ T cells in patients with idiopathic thrombocytopenic purpura. *Thromb. Res.* 2007,120:187-193.
[132] Liu, M. F., Wang, C. R., Fung, L. L., Wu, C. R. Decreased CD4+CD25+ T cells in peripheral blood of patients with systemic lupus erythematosus. *Scand. J. Immunol.* 2004,59:198-202.

[133] Furuno, K., Yuge, T., Kusuhara, K., Takada, H., Nishio, H., Khajoee, V., et al. CD25+CD4+ regulatory T cells in patients with Kawasaki disease. *J. Pediatr.* 2004,145:385-390.

[134] Chi, L. J., Wang, H. B., Zhang, Y., Wang, W. Z. Abnormality of circulating CD4(+)CD25(+) regulatory T cell in patients with Guillain-Barre syndrome. *J. Neuroimmunol.* 2007,192:206-214.

[135] Brusko, T. M., Wasserfall, C. H., Clare-Salzler, M. J., Schatz, D. A., Atkinson, M. A. Functional defects and the influence of age on the frequency of CD4+ CD25+ T-cells in type 1 diabetes. *Diabetes* 2005, 54: 1407-1414.

[136] Lindley, S., Dayan, C. M., Bishop, A., Roep, B. O., Peakman, M., Tree, T. I. Defective suppressor function in CD4(+)CD25(+) T-cells from patients with type 1 diabetes. *Diabetes* 2005,54:92-99.

[137] Haas, J., Hug, A., Viehover, A., Fritzsching, B., Falk, C. S., Filser, A., et al. Reduced suppressive effect of CD4+CD25high regulatory T cells on the T cell immune response against myelin oligodendrocyte glycoprotein in patients with multiple sclerosis. *Eur. J. Immunol.* 2005,35:3343-3352.

[138] Viglietta, V., Baecher-Allan, C., Weiner, H. L., Hafler, D. A. Loss of functional suppression by CD4+CD25+ regulatory T cells in patients with multiple sclerosis. *J. Exp. Med.* 2004,199:971-979.

[139] Olivito, B., Taddio, A., Simonini, G., Massai, C., Ciullini, S., Gambineri, E., et al. Defective FOXP3 expression in patients with acute Kawasaki disease and restoration by intravenous immunoglobulin therapy. *Clin. Exp. Rheumatol.* 2010,28:93-97.

[140] Tsurikisawa, N., Saito, H., Oshikata, C., Tsuburai, T., Akiyama, K. High-dose intravenous immunoglobulin treatment increases regulatory T cells in patients with eosinophilic granulomatosis with polyangiitis. *J. Rheumatol.* 2012,39:1019-1025.

[141] Bayry, J., Mouthon, L., Kaveri, S. V. Intravenous immunoglobulin expands regulatory T cells in autoimmune rheumatic disease. *J. Rheumatol.* 2012,39:450-451.

[142] Ephrem, A., Chamat, S., Miquel, C., Fisson, S., Mouthon, L., Caligiuri, G., et al. Expansion of CD4+CD25+ regulatory T cells by intravenous immunoglobulin: a critical factor in controlling experimental auto-immune encephalomyelitis. *Blood* 2008,111:715-722.

[143] Ramakrishna, C., Newo, A. N., Shen, Y. W., Cantin, E. Passively administered pooled human immunoglobulins exert IL-10 dependent anti-inflammatory effects that protect against fatal HSV encephalitis. *PLoS Pathog.* 2011,7:e1002071.

[144] Massoud, A. H., Guay, J., Shalaby, K. H., Bjur, E., Ablona, A., Chan, D., et al. Intravenous immunoglobulin attenuates airway inflammation through induction of forkhead box protein 3-positive regulatory T cells. *J. Allergy Clin. Immunol.* 2012,129:1656-1665 e1653.
[145] Kessel, A., Ammuri, H., Peri, R., Pavlotzky, E. R., Blank, M., Shoenfeld, Y., et al. Intravenous immunoglobulin therapy affects T regulatory cells by increasing their suppressive function. *J. Immunol.* 2007,179:5571-5575.
[146] Tha-In, T., Metselaar, H. J., Bushell, A. R., Kwekkeboom, J., Wood, K. J. Intravenous immunoglobulins promote skin allograft acceptance by triggering functional activation of CD4+Foxp3+ T cells. *Transplantation* 2010,89:1446-1455.
[147] Massoud, A. H., Yona, M., Xue, D., Chouiali, F., Alturaihi, H., Ablona, A., et al. Dendritic cell immunoreceptor: A novel receptor for intravenous immunoglobulin mediates induction of regulatory T cells. *J. Allergy Clin. Immunol.* 2013.
[148] Trinath, J., Hegde, P., Sharma, M., Maddur, M. S., Rabin, M., Vallat, J. M., et al. Intravenous immunoglobulin expands regulatory T cells via induction of cyclooxygenase-2-dependent prostaglandin E2 in human dendritic cells. *Blood* 2013,122:1419-1427.
[149] De Groot, A. S., Moise, L., McMurry, J. A., Wambre, E., Van Overtvelt, L., Moingeon, P., et al. Activation of natural regulatory T cells by IgG Fc-derived peptide "Tregitopes". *Blood* 2008,112:3303-3311.
[150] Cousens, L. P., Su, Y., McClaine, E., Li, X., Terry, F., Smith, R., et al. Application of IgG-derived natural Treg epitopes (IgG Tregitopes) to antigen-specific tolerance induction in a murine model of type 1 diabetes. *J. Diabetes Res.* 2013,2013:621693.
[151] Van der Marel, S., Majowicz, A., Kwikkers, K., van Logtenstein, R., te Velde, A. A., De Groot, A. S., et al. Adeno-associated virus mediated delivery of Tregitope 167 ameliorates experimental colitis. *World J. Gastroenterol.* 2012,18:4288-4299.
[152] Paquin Proulx, D., Aubin, E., Lemieux, R., Bazin, R. Inhibition of B cell-mediated antigen presentation by intravenous immunoglobulins (IVIg). *Clin. Immunol.* 2010,135:422-429.
[153] Proulx, D. P., Aubin, E., Lemieux, R., Bazin, R. Spontaneous internalization of IVIg in activated B cells. *Immunol. Lett.* 2009,124:18-26.
[154] Cousens, L. P., Tassone, R., Mazer, B. D., Ramachandiran, V., Scott, D. W., De Groot, A. S. Tregitope update: mechanism of action parallels IVIg. *Autoimmun. Rev.* 2013,12:436-443.

[155] Elyaman, W., Khoury, S. J., Scott, D. W., De Groot, A. S. Potential application of tregitopes as immunomodulating agents in multiple sclerosis. *Neurol. Res. Int.* 2011,2011:256460.

[156] Yen, H. R., Harris, T. J., Wada, S., Grosso, J. F., Getnet, D., Goldberg, M. V., et al. Tc17 CD8 T cells: functional plasticity and subset diversity. *J. Immunol.* 2009,183:7161-7168.

[157] Wang, Y. M., Alexander, S. I. CD8 regulatory T cells: what's old is now new. *Immunol. Cell Biol.* 2009,87:192-193.

[158] Anikeeva, N., Sykulev, Y. Mechanisms controlling granule-mediated cytolytic activity of cytotoxic T lymphocytes. *Immunol. Res.* 2011,51: 183-194.

[159] Lieberman, J. The ABCs of granule-mediated cytotoxicity: new weapons in the arsenal. *Nat. Rev. Immunol.* 2003,3:361-370.

[160] Mosmann, T. R., Li, L., Sad, S. Functions of CD8 T-cell subsets secreting different cytokine patterns. *Semin. Immunol.* 1997,9:87-92.

[161] Walter, U., Santamaria, P. CD8+ T cells in autoimmunity. *Curr. Opin. Immunol.* 2005,17:624-631.

[162] Korber, J., Kottgen, E., Renz, H. A case of Crohn's disease with increased CD8 T-cell activation and remission during therapy with intravenous immunoglobulins. *Scand. J. Gastroenterol.* 1998,33:1113-1117.

[163] Mausberg, A. K., Dorok, M., Stettner, M., Muller, M., Hartung, H. P., Dehmel, T., et al. Recovery of the T-cell repertoire in CIDP by IV immunoglobulins. *Neurology* 2013,80:296-303.

[164] Trepanier, P., Chabot, D., Bazin, R. Intravenous immunoglobulin modulates the expansion and cytotoxicity of CD8(+) T cells. *Immunology* 2014,141:233-241.

[165] Hogquist, K. A., Jameson, S. C., Heath, W. R., Howard, J. L., Bevan, M. J., Carbone, F. R. T cell receptor antagonist peptides induce positive selection. *Cell* 1994,76:17-27.

[166] Trepanier, P., Bazin, R. Intravenous immunoglobulin (IVIg) inhibits CD8 cytotoxic T-cell activation. *Blood* 2012,120:2769-2770.

[167] Misra, N., Bayary, J., Dasgupta, S., Ephrem, A., Huyen, J. P., Delignat, S., et al. Intravenous immunoglobulin and dendritic cells. *Clin. Rev. Allergy Immunol.* 2005,29:201-205.

In: Plasmapheresis and Intravenous … ISBN: 978-1-63117-916-7
Editor: Rossana Allegro

Chapter 5

INTRAVENOUS IMMUNOGLOBIN (IVIG): CLINICAL USES IN AUTOIMMUNE DISORDERS AS ESPECIALLY EOSINOPHILIC GRANULOMATOSIS WITH POLYANGIITIS, POTENTIAL COMPLICATIONS AND LONG-TERM EFFICACY

Naomi Tsurikisawa, MD*[*1], Hiroshi Saito, PhD[2], Chiyako Oshikata, MD[1] and Kazuo Akiyama[1, 2]

[1]Departments of Allergy and Respirology and
[2]the Clinical Research Center for Allergy and Rheumatology,
National Hospital Organization, Sagamihara National Hospital,
Minami-ku Sagamihara, Kanagawa, Japan

ABSTRACT

Eosinophilic granulomatosis with polyangiitis (EGPA; also known as Churg–Strauss Syndrome) is a rare disease characterized by allergic granulomatosis and necrotizing vasculitis following peripheral and tissue eosinophilia. The mortality and prognosis associated with EGPA are related to disease severity, as assessed by Five-Factor Scores; the survival

---

[*] Corresponding author's email; n-tsurikisawa@sagamihara-hosp.gr.jp

rate at 5 years after myocardial involvement is reported to be one-third of that without myocardial involvement.

The mainstay of treatment for EGPA is systemic corticosteroid (CS) therapy. Additional treatments with immunosuppressive agents such as cyclophosphamide (CYC) or azathioprine may be helpful in some patients. However, mononeuritis multiplex or heart failure in some patients with EGPA or with antineutrophil cytoplasmic autoantibody (ANCA)-associated systemic vasculitis does not respond to combination therapy.

High-dose intravenous immunoglobulin (IVIG) therapy was effective against severe mononeuritis multiplex or heart failure in patients with EGPA that did not respond to combination therapy. IVIG treatment has thus shown clinical efficacy; it regulates the activation of T_{reg} cells in autoimmune and immune-mediated inflammatory diseases. Mechanisms implicated in IVIG modulation of T_{reg} function include activation and induction of T_{reg} cells by the Fc or $F(ab')_2$ domain of IVIG and enhancement of T_{reg} function by increasing the expression of FOXP3, TGF-β, IL-10, and CTLA-4. We confirmed that the number of T_{reg} cells is increased for at least two years after the last IVIG treatment. This finding could lead to a reduction in the maintenance dose of CS and suggests that IVIG therapy may improve the prognosis of EGPA patients with severe organ involvement.

However administration of IVIG alone, without concomitant treatment with CS and CYC as an initial treatment approach for EGPA, did not improve pulmonary infiltration or vasculitic symptoms in various organs, including the digestive tract and skin. Furthermore, it had no effect on peripheral nerve damage, cardiac dysfunction, or eosinophil numbers (including $CD69^+CCR3^+$-activated eosinophils). Moreover, it is unclear whether the clinical and immunologic efficacy of IVIG is affected by the disease phase (e.g., during initial treatment or at relapse after remission). In addition, the characteristics of the patient's disease condition that influence whether remission is achieved after a single course or multiple courses of IVIG have not been assessed.

INTRODUCTION

Eosinophilic granulomatosis with polyangiitis (EGPA; also known as Churg-Strauss syndrome) is a rare disease characterized by the presence of allergic granulomatosis and necrotizing vasculitis. Development of the condition is preceded by peripheral blood eosinophilia and eosinophilic tissue infiltration [1]. EGPA is classified as a vasculitis of arteries that are small to medium in diameter, although such vasculitis is often not apparent in the initial phases of the disease [2].

Before the development of corticosteroids (CS), the mortality rate of patients with EGPA was approximately 50% within 3 months of diagnosis [3, 4]. The 5-year survival rate was 62%–79% [3, 5–7]. The prognosis of EGPA patients, and the extent of mortality from the disease, are associated with disease severity, as assessed by using the Five-Factor Scores (FFSs) developed in 1996 [7] and 2009 [8]. In addition, myocardial involvement [4] and the presence of gastrointestinal disease [4, 9] are independent negative prognostic factors. The remission rate after initial treatment is reported to be 81% to 91% in EGPA patients. This may be compared with the 30% to 93% remission rate in patients with granulomatosis polyangiitis (GPA, known as Wegener's granulomatosis) and the 75% to 89% remission rate in those with microscopic polyangiitis (MPA) [10]. However, the relapse rate is higher in EGPA patients in the first 2 years after diagnosis than in MPA patients (35% in EGPA patients vs. 8% in those with MPA [10]). The relapse rate in EGPA patients after 5 years or more is greater than 60%, compared with 20% in MPA patients [11]. Moreover, the relapse rate of EGPA patients with FFS = 0 or 1 is 35% during the first year of treatment [12].

Clinical Manifestations

EGPA is a rare disorder characterized by an incidence of 0.11 to 2.66 new cases per million population per year and an overall prevalence of 10.7 to 14 per 1,000,000 adults [13–15]. The male-to-female ratio ranges from 0.3 to 2.3 and the mean age at onset varies from 38 to 52 years (range, 7–74 years) [16, 17]. Nonetheless, there is a generally agreed-upon clinical description of the disease. The frequencies of organ involvement and other clinical features of EGPA previously reported by others and observed at our hospital are summarized in Table 1 [18]. EGPA is usually induced in anti-neutrophil cytoplasmic antibody (ANCA)-associated vasculitis, GPA, and MPA. The prevalence of ANCA in EGPA is less consistent than that of GPA or MPA. Myeloperoxidase (MPO) - ANCA was positive at a rate of approximately 40% of EGPA, compared with 50-80% of MPA. Proteinase 3 (PR3-ANCA) whereas was rare in EGPA, compared with positively rate of >90%. GPA [4][17][19][16][20][21].

Table I. Clinical manifestations of vasculitis

	Churg	Chumbley	Lanham	Hashimoto	Guillevin	Sagamihara
	U.S.	U.S.	U.K.	Japan	France	Japan
	1951	1977	1984	1994	1999	2011 and 2012
Cases	13	30	138	87	96	86
M/F	4/9	21/9	72/66	41/46	45/51	27/59
Mean age (y)	33	47	38	47	48	53.4
Age range (y)	(7–62)	(15–69)		(17–79)	(17–74)	(19–83)
Clinical manifestations (%)						
Asthma	100	100	100	93	100	100
Pulmonary infiltrates	39	27	74	33	38	80
Sinusitis	77	70	69		48	91
Multiplex mononeuritis	69	63	64	65	78	99
Gastrointestinal	92	17	62	19	33	85
Heart	54	16	52	33	30	74
Arthritis	31	20	46	52	41	42
Myalgias			33	51	54	25
Skin		66	51			
Purpura	62		46	44	31	67
Nodules	54	27	33	27	19	6
Renal	31	20	46	46	16	58
Central nervous system	61		27		8	18

Recently, it was shown that different clinical phenotypes could be observed according to the presence or absence of ANCA, thereby suggesting that different disease mechanisms are involved in the pathogenesis of EGPA. Increased prevalence of central nervous system involvement [22], renal involvement, peripheral neuropathy, and pulmonary hemorrhage [23] has been reported among ANCA-positive patients. Negative ANCA status is associated with heart disease and lung involvement [23]. From these findings, it has been hypothesized that, as in GPA and MPA, ANCAs may contribute directly to the endothelial vasculitic damage seen in ANCA-positive patients, whereas in ANCA-negative patients, eosinophils may be directly responsible for the release of cationic proteins and eosinophil-derived neurotoxin [24]. These data suggest that EGPA, when presenting as a form of necrotizing small-vessel vasculitis, is a true ANCA-associated disease, characterized by positivity for MPO-ANCAs. Alternatively, ANCA-negative patients may be clinically characterized by tissue infiltration by eosinophils that results in fibrotic organ damage; their disease may belong more to the spectrum of hypereosinophilic syndromes rather than to the spectrum of ANCA vasculitis. The existence of two clinical phenotypes may reveal different pathways of pathogenicity in EGPA.

Asthma is present in 96% to 100% of EGPA patients and is the cardinal feature of EGPA. Asthma may precede systemic vasculitis by approximately 8 years and, in some cases, by more than 30 years [1, 6, 4, 25]. The precise etiology of EGPA and the asthmatic phase that precedes it, as well as the role of genetic factors, remains unknown. In our retrospective cohort study, we found that the clinical manifestations of asthma occur in the pre-vasculitic phase of the disease [26]. The asthma of 87.5% of 24 patients in the pre-vasculitic phase of EGPA at their first hospital visit was severe. It was characterized in 42.9% of these patients as requiring treatment with systemic steroids and mechanical ventilation and by the presence of sinusitis in 57.1% of these patients during the period from the first hospital visit to the onset of EGPA (Table II) [26]. The percentage of eosinophils in the peripheral blood of pre-EGPA asthmatics at the first hospital visit was also significantly higher than that in non-EGPA asthmatics ($p < 0.01$). The percentage of eosinophils in the peripheral blood could be used to predict future onset of EGPA with reasonably high specificity (99.4%) and high sensitivity (66.7%), with a cut-off point of 20% [26]. The percentage forced expiratory volume (%FEV1) in the severe asthmatics and the asthmatic patients who later developed EGPA was lower than that in patients with mild or moderate asthma. The %FEV1 in the asthmatic patients who later developed EGPA was the same as that in patients with severe asthma. However, bronchial hyperresponsiveness to acetylcholine in the pre-vasculitic patients was significantly less severe than that in the non-EGPA patients with severe asthma and was as mild as that in patients with mild asthma [26]. Thus, asthma severity in the pre-vasculitic phase of EGPA is related to airflow limitation and to eosinophilic inflammation in the peripheral blood but not to bronchial hyperresponsiveness, which may occur as a result of airway vasculitis. We propose that asthma patients who develop EGPA differ from other asthma patients, from whom they can be differentiated at the first hospital visit by evaluating these factors.

Table II. Differences between patients with non-EGPA (also known as Churg-Strauss syndrome) severe asthma, and those with severe asthma in the pre-vasculitic phase of EGPA. (Modified, with permission, from Tsurikisawa et al. [26])

Characteristics	General asthmatics severe asthma N = 130 (44.2%)	Before EGPA severe asthma N = 21 (85.5%)	*P*-value
Systemic corticosteroid	N = 9 (6.9%)	N = 9 (42.9%)	$P < 0.0001$
mg: converted to the prednisolone equivalent	5.3 ± 2.0	7.2 ± 3.6	N.S.
ICS (μg: converted to the beclomethasone equivalent)	1194.7 ± 575.1	1371.4 ± 721.9	N.S.
Intubation	N = 2(1.5%)	N = 3 (14.3%)	$P = 0.0018$
Sinusitis	N = 40 (30.8%)	N = 12 (57.1%)	$P < 0.0001$
CEP	N = 3 (2.3%)	N = 7 (33.3%)	$P < 0.0001$

Mean ± SD.
Comparison were made by using the X^2 Test.
ICS; inhaled corticosteroid.
CEP; chronic eosinophilic pneumonia.
N.S.; not significant.

MECHANISMS

Eosinophilic infiltrations, such as those found in chronic eosinophilic pneumonia (CEP) and eosinophilic gastroenteritis, precede systemic vasculitis in half of all patients with EGPA [25][27]. Some clinicians believe that patients with CEP after asthma are more likely to develop EGPA if the CEP is left untreated. However, some patients in whom asthma is complicated by CEP do not develop EGPA. There is no clear mechanism that explains why some CEP patients with asthma develop EGPA, yet others do not. The etiology of idiopathic CEP is not understood, although in some cases CEP is caused by infection with a parasite, virus, or fungus or by drugs, toxic agents, or radiation therapy. Asthma occurs before CEP in about one-half to two-thirds of CEP patients [28, 29]. Increasing numbers of eosinophils and lymphocytes in the peripheral blood and bronchoalveolar lavage fluid (BALF) contribute to the development of CEP. There are many mediators of eosinophilia in CEP, including regulated upon activation normal T-cell-expressed and -secreted (RANTES), eotaxin, thymus- and activation-regulated chemokine (TARC/CCL17), and cytokines, including IL-2, IL-3, IL-5, IL-10, IL-13, and IL-18. The number of $CD4^{+}CD25^{+}$ T cells in the BALF and peripheral blood is increased in patients with CEP [30]. By contrast, peripheral blood mononuclear cells in patients with EGPA secrete not only the type 1 cytokine IFN-γ, but also type 2 cytokines, such as IL-4, IL-13, and, in particular, IL-5. The number of $CD4^{+}CD25^{+}$ T cells producing IL-5, which causes eosinophilia in peripheral blood cells and lung tissue, is high in EGPA and CEP patients at disease onset and decreases significantly after the EGPA is treated and the CEP resolves [31].

Regulatory T (T_{reg}) cells play central roles in the maintenance of both immune homeostasis and peripheral tolerance. Naturally occurring $CD4^{+}$ regulatory T (nT_{reg}) cells constitutively express the proteins forkhead box P (FOXP)3 and CD25. T_{reg} cells may also be identified by co-expression, on the cell surface, of cytotoxic T-lymphocyte antigen-4 (CTLA-4), CD25, and CD4. Natural T_{reg} cells suppress autoimmune T cell responses and maintain peripheral tolerance by preventing the differentiation of T_{reg} cells into effector T cells [32] Peripheral differentiation of inducible T_{reg} (iT_{reg}) cells, which secrete IL-10, requires high-level T-cell-receptor signaling, an elevated level of serum TGF-β, and expression of IL-10 [33]. When TGF-β mediates induction of iT_{reg} cells, CTLA-4 must bind to either the co-stimulatory B7 family molecule CD80 or CD86 [34]. Recent studies have focused on T_{reg} cells and the mechanisms of human autoimmune or inflammatory diseases.[35-40] However, whether T_{reg} cell activity is involved in the mechanism and etiology of EGPA is not known. We examined the phenotypes and functions of $CD4^{+}CD25^{+}$ T cells from asthma patients with CEP and from EGPA patients at disease onset and after therapy and then compared our findings with those in patients with general asthma. We found that, at disease onset, EGPA patients, unlike CEP patients, had significantly fewer $CD4^{+}CD25^{+}$ T cells than did patients with any type of asthma (steps 1–4) [31, 41]. $CD4^{+}CD25^{+}$ T cells that produced IL-10 were rarely detected in EGPA patients at disease onset or relapse, whereas the numbers of IL-10–producing T cells in CEP patients were high at disease onset. Fewer $CD4^{+}CD25^{-}$ T cells producing IL-2 were found in EGPA patients before treatment than were found in CEP patients at disease onset. The proportions of $CD4^{+}CD25^{+}$ T cells producing IL-10 and of $CD4^{+}CD25^{-}$ T cells producing IL-2 in EGPA patients significantly increased at remission after treatment. We thus confirmed that maintenance of T_{reg} cell numbers in asthma patients with CEP may inhibit EGPA development via the action of cytokines, such as IL-10 and IL-2, produced by $CD4^{+}CD25^{+}$ and $CD4^{+}CD25^{-}$ T cells, respectively [31].

Th17 cells are CD4 T cells that are characterized by the production of IL-17A, IL-17F, and IL-22, which have been implicated in the pathogenesis of protective immunity against some bacterial infections, mainly through the recruitment and activation of neutrophils, and of several autoimmune diseases [42]. Th17 cells play important roles in the immune response depending on their stage of differentiation, be it induction, amplification, or stabilization. In mice, TGF-β induces the development of inducible T_{reg} cells by inducing the expression of the transcription factor Foxp-3 and the production IL-17A by CD4 T cells. IL-6, IL-1β, TNF-α, and IL-21, together with TGF-β, promote Th17 differentiation or polarization. IL-6 promotes induction of the nuclear receptor retinoic acid-related orphan receptor γt (RORγt) and suppresses the differentiation of T_{reg} cells. IL-2 suppresses the differentiation of Th17 cells. Foxp3 T_{reg} cells suppress the activation of the transcription factor for RORγt by binding directly to RORγt [43]. In mice, IL-17 increases after a decrease in Foxp-3 expression induced by the induction of IL-6 or IL-1 [44]. Some reports have suggested that Th17 cells are related to vasculitis, such as Takayasu's arteritis [45], giant cell arteritis [46], Henoch-Schönlein purpura [47], ANCA-associated vasculitis [48, 49], GPA/WG [50], and EGPA/CSS [51, 52].

We confirmed that the percentage of $CD4^{+}$ T cells producing IL-17 was significantly greater in patients with active EGPA than in healthy control patients or in patients with asthma, CEP, or inactive EGPA ($p < 0.01$) [52]. Moreover, the percentage of $CD4^{+}$ T cells producing IL-17 in patients with active EGPA who were at onset or at relapse was significantly greater than that in patients with inactive EGPA, and the percentage of $CD4^{+}CD25^{+}$ T cells producing IL-10 (Tr1 cells) in patients with active EGPA was significantly smaller than that in patients with inactive EGPA who achieved remission after treatment (Tr 1) [52]. Th17 cells were identified as $CD4^{+}$ T cells that produce mainly IL-17 and IL-22. As stated earlier, eosinophilia is a characteristic of EGPA, and some reports suggest that the IL-25 produced by eosinophils promotes innate adaptive immunity by enhancing Th2 cytokine production [53]. We showed that the number of $CD4^{+}$ T cells producing IL-17 or IL-22 in the peripheral blood of EGPA patients increases at relapse and that the numbers of these $CD4^{+}$ T cells correlate with the number of $CD4^{+}$ T cells producing IL-25 [54]. Indoleamine 2, 3-dioxygenase (IDO) expression in monocytes from all EGPA patients is positively correlated with the percentage of $CD4^+CD25^+$ T_{reg} cells producing IL-10 and inversely correlated with the percentage of Th17 cells. Thus EGPA relapse may be linked to elevated levels of IL-25 producing $CD4^+$ T cells, which promotes Th2 inflammation and reduce Tr1 cell subpopulations, which also result from lower IDO expression in monocytes. Thus, the percentages of $CD4^+CD25^+$ T_{reg} cells producing IL-10 and of Th17 cells reflect the disease activity of EGPA [52]. IL-27 is known to antagonize Th17 development, induce IL-10 production, and suppress IL-6-induced T cell proliferation [55]. We confirmed that an increase in IL-27 production by $CD14^+$ monocytes and a decrease in the percentage of $CD14^+$ monocytes producing IL-23p19 induces differentiation of $CD4^+CD25^+$ T_{reg} cells producing IL-10 and suppresses differentiation of Th17 cells in EGPA patients in remission [56].

The relapse rate is higher for EGPA patients than for MPA patients; some patients with EGPA experience frequent relapses after initial clinical remission, whereas others fail to enter remission that lasts for extended periods. The mechanisms underlying the intractable form of EGPA remain poorly understood. In our studies, frequently relapsing EGPA patients, defined as patients who relapse at least once every 2 years after an initial period of remission, exhibited decreased T_{reg} cell counts and increased percentages of B cells that scored as $CD80^+$, $CD27^+$, or $CD95^+$. Patients with frequently relapsing EGPA had increased percentages of $CD27^+$ and $CD95^+$ B cells, and fewer $CD19^+$ B cells, than did patients in the other seldom relapsing groups. Lower $CD19^+$ B cell counts were associated with reduced T_{reg} cell counts and a lower serum IgG concentration. In patients with frequently relapsing EGPA, decreases in T_{reg} cell numbers and increased percentages of activated B cells may induce apoptosis of B cells [57].

TREATMENT

The mainstay of treatment for EGPA is systemic corticosteroids (CS) therapy. Additional treatment with immunosuppressive agents, such as cyclophosphamide (CYC) or azathioprine, may be of benefit to some patients. Other treatment options [58] include methotrexate, mycophenolate mofetil, rituximab, interferon-α, anti-IgE therapy, anti-IL-5 antibodies, anti-TNF-α (infliximab, etanercept, adalimumab), plasma exchange, and intravenous immunoglobulin (IVIG). Corticosteroids and immunosuppressants, especially CYC, have considerably improved most symptoms of vasculitis, particularly those involving the gastrointestinal system, skin, and lungs, as well as constitutional symptoms. However mononeuritis multiplex and heart failure in patients with EGPA or ANCA-associated systemic vasculitis do not respond to combination therapy with CS and CYC; paralysis, presenting as multiple mononeuropathy, often remains [59–62].

Rehabilitation for multiple mononeuropathy is as important for EGPA patients as their therapeutic management [63]. Because patients with mononeuritis multiplex have restricted weakness in the muscles ruled by specific nerves and functional improvement may be gradual, rehabilitation approaches, including orthoses, are of value to improve the compensatory ability of the normal adjacent muscles even in the early stages of the treatment [64]. We found that the application of transdermal isosorbide dinitrate (ISDN) patches to the toes of the affected leg or hand produces warming and decreases numbness. The application of ISDN patches also increased the skin temperature, not only on the affected side of the leg or hand but also on the contralateral site [65]. The mechanism involves an increase in blood flow, via local and systemic vasodilating effects, in the region where the ISDN patches are applied; this increased blood flow reduces hyperalgesia and blocks neurogenic inflammation, leading to improved nerve conduction by increasing neuronal postsynaptic cyclic GNP levels.

IVIG therapy has been used to treat various diseases, including MPA, GPA, and ANCA-associated systemic vasculitis at initial treatment [66–68]. And IVIGs induced complete remissions of relapsed ANCA-associated vasculitides [69]. Hamilos et al. [70] were the first to report that eosinophilia in EGPA is improved by treatment with IVIG; other investigators have since described successful treatment with IVIG of EGPA itself [71, 72]. We previously reported that IVIG therapy improved mononeuritis multiplex or heart failure in 14 of 15 patients with EGPA who did not respond to combination therapy with CS and CYC. IVIG (dosed at 400 mg per kg per day) was given daily for 5 days [73]. Neuropathy was evaluated by assessing manual muscle strength and skin temperature at affected sites. Cardiac function was evaluated by using ejection fraction assessment with echocardiography and two imaging tests of the myocardium (^{123}I-meta-iodobenzylguanidine (MIBG) and ^{201}Tl). We found that manual muscle strength improved and that the skin temperature of both hands and legs significantly increased on IVIG therapy. In the five patients with heart failure, the ejection fraction of the left ventricle significantly increased from 35.2% to 61.0%. Myocardial uptake of ^{123}MIBG significantly increased, indicating improved myocardial viability. ^{201}Tl images showed a perfusion defect and that following IVIG therapy, blood perfusion improved. IVIG therapy may induce remission by ameliorating neuropathy and heart failure in patients who are unresponsive to treatment with CS or CYC.

However, administration of IVIG alone, without concomitant treatment with CSs and CYC as an initial treatment approach for EGPA, did not improve pulmonary infiltration or vasculitic symptoms in various organs, including the digestive tract and skin [18]. IVIG should, therefore, not be used in place of conventional therapy with CSs or immunosuppressants such as CYC, except when patients are resistant to such therapy [74].

MECHANISMS OF ACTION OF IVIG

Multiple mechanisms have been proposed for the action of IVIG in autoimmune or systemic inflammatory disease, and they involve numerous components of the immune system, including: 1) Fc receptors (blockade of Fc receptors on macrophages and effector cells, induction of antibody-dependent cellular cytotoxicity or inhibitory Fcγ receptor IIB); 2) inflammation (attenuation of complement-mediated tissue damage, reduction of immune-complex-mediated inflammation, induction of anti-inflammatory cytokines, inhibition of activation of endothelial cells, neutralization of microbial toxins, and reduction in corticosteroid requirements); 3) B cells and antibodies (control of emergent bone marrow B cell repertoires, negative signaling through Fcγ receptors, selective down-regulation and up-regulation of antibody production, neutralization of circulating autoantibodies by antiidiotypes, and modulation of immunoglobulin production or long-term modification of antibody repertoires); 4) T cells (regulation of the production of helper-T-cell cytokines, and neutralization of T-cell superantigens); and 5) cell growth (inhibition of lymphocyte proliferation, and regulation of apoptosis) [75, 76]. The Fc region of IVIG induces the activation and induction of T_{reg} cells via the increased expression of Foxp3, TGF-β, IL-10, and cytotoxic T-lymphocyte antigen-4 (CTLA-4) with enhanced functions [77–80]. These effects of IVIG on T_{reg} cells may be mediated by direct the interaction of self-reactive natural autoantibodies with T cell surface molecules [75][81] and the suppression of allogeneic T-cell responses through direct activation of T_{reg} cells [82]. The conserved T cell epitopes derived from the Fc region (Tregitopes) can induce and activate T_{reg} cells via the expression of $CD25^{high}$ or CTLA-4 [78]. Sialic acid crystallizable fragments (sFc) on IgG bind to DC-SIGN on dendritic cells and induce IL-33 production, which in turn, induces expansion of IL-4–producing basophils that promote increased expression of the inhibitory Fc receptor (FcγRIIB) on effector macrophages [83]. IVIG inhibits the differentiation and amplification of Th17 cells, as well as the production of their effector cytokines IL-17A, IL-17F, IL-21, and CCL20 [84]. The inhibitory effects of IVIG on Th17 cells are F(ab′)-dependent and involve interference with the expression of RORγt. Sialic acid-positive IgG binding with CD22 promotes apoptosis in mature B cells through B cell receptor signaling [85].

We examined the long-term efficacy of IVIG in patients with EGPA. EGPA patients with severe multiple mononeuritis or cardiac dysfunction received IVIG therapy in combination with conventional therapy. As a control, EGPA patients without severe vasculitic symptoms were treated with conventional therapy and without IVIG. Multiple mononeuritis and cardiac dysfunction improved after immunoglobulin therapy and the maintenance corticosteroid dose was lower than that for the controls. The frequencies of T_{reg} cells, defined as $CD25^{+}CD4^{+}$ T cells producing IL-10, and of $FOXP3^{+}CD4^{+}$ T cells in the peripheral blood were lower at onset in the study group than in the control patients. However, relative to the controls, the numbers of these cells increased significantly over an extended period after the last immunoglobulin dose [86]. This finding led to a reduction of the amount of corticosteroids needed [86]. Several other authors have also reported that IVIG treatment may reduce the amount of corticosteroids needed for maintenance of remission of EGPA [87]. We expect that IVIG for frequently relapsing EGPA patients may reconstitute B cell function by increasing T_{reg} cells and IgG in serum.

We also examined the effect of IVIG on peripheral eosinophil counts and CD69 expression on the surfaces of eosinophils. IVIG therapy did not affect the peripheral blood eosinophil count, but it did downregulate the expression of CD69. This finding suggests that, in EGPA, activated eosinophils survive even after CS or CYC treatment, and that IVIG therapy decreases the number of activated eosinophils that express early activation markers such as CD69. The progression of EGPA may, therefore, be related more to the abundance of CD69-expressing eosinophils than to the total number of eosinophils. Anti-sialic acid–binding Ig-like lectin-8 autoantibodies present in IVIG have been reported to promote apoptosis of eosinophils [88]. Thus, one mechanism by which IVIG therapy acts on EGPA may be via the inactivation of eosinophils [73].

Furthermore, IVIG therapy without administration of CS had no effect on peripheral nerve damage, cardiac dysfunction, the number of eosinophils (including $CD69^+CCR3^+$-activated eosinophils), or the proportion of eosinophils with vacuole formation [18]. This suggests that CS administration reduces eosinophil counts but does not reduce the percentage of activated eosinophils, and that IVIG administered with CSs may exhibit an adjuvant effect.

However, whether the clinical and immunologic efficacy of IVIG is affected by disease phase (e.g., if given as part of initial treatment or at relapse after remission) is unknown. The characteristics of the patient's disease condition that influence whether remission is achieved after a single course or multiple courses of IVIG had not previously been assessed. We evaluated whether the frequency of T_{reg} cells varied depending on when IVIG was provided after the start of conventional therapy for EGPA. $FOXP3^+CD4^+$ T cell numbers increased in patients who required only a single course of IVIG to achieve remission compared with those needed at least two courses. The dosage of prednisolone at initial IVIG treatment was inversely correlated with the ratio between the number of $FOXP3^+CD4^+$ T cells before and that at 1 month thereafter. T_{reg} cell numbers at one month after IVIG failed to increase in more than half of the patients given prednisolone doses exceeding 40 mg during IVIG treatment, and high-dose prednisolone may have suppressed the serum IgG levels [89]. Many inflammatory mediators are present in various quantities in serum during the acute disease associated with the initial treatment of EGPA; these mediators might therefore out-compete IVIG and suppress the differentiation of T_{reg} cells. An increase in T_{reg} cell frequency after IVIG administration may predict the need for more IVIG in EGPA.

Prognosis

Before the use of CSs, the mortality rate for EGPA was approximately 50% within 3 months of diagnosis [3, 4]. Other reports suggest a 5-year survival rate for EGPA of 62% to 80% [3, 5–7]. Most deaths result from complications of the vasculitic phase of the disease and are due to cardiac failure or myocardial infarction, cerebral hemorrhage, renal failure, gastrointestinal bleeding, or status asthmaticus. The presence or absence of the features that make up the five-factor score (FFS2009) [age > 65 years, cardiac involvement, gastrointestinal disease (bleeding, perforation, infarction, or pancreatitis), and renal insufficiency (creatinine concentration >1.5 mg/dl)] has been used to predict survival in EGPA [8]. The 5, 10, and 20-year mortality rates were about 90%, 75%, and 45%, respectively, reported in 2011 by Guillevin et al. and 97%, 89%, and 72% respectively, reported in 2013 by Moosing et al. [90]. The prognosis and mortality rates have improved as a result of improved diagnosis in accordance with American Collage of Rheumatology (ACR) criteria from 1994 and improvements in appropriate treatments over the last twenty years.

The remission rate for EGPA ranges from 81% to 91% and the relapse rate ranges from 20% to 60% [10, 11]. Gastrointestinal involvement, persistent ANCA positivity, and a rise in ANCA titer are all risk factors for relapse. We reported that cardiac sympathetic nerve function is damaged in EGPA patients with cardiac involvement and that ^{123}I-MIBG scintigraphy is useful for detecting cardiac involvement and predicting relapse due to cardiac events [91].

CONCLUSION

The prognosis for EGPA, evaluated on the basis of a 5- or 10-year survival rate, has improved since 2000. Diagnostic skills have progressed, as have early intervention treatments with steroids and other additional therapeutic immunosuppressive agents. IVIG therapy for EGPA patients has improved clinical symptoms due to vasculitis, such as multiplex mononeuritis or cardiac dysfunction, and decreased the need for systemic CS intake by increasing T_{reg} cell numbers or decreasing activated CD69-positive eosinophils. The use of IVIG, in addition to conventional treatment for EGPA, has been widespread in Japan because IVIG has been covered by insurance since Jan 2010. We believe that IVIG may reconstruct B cell function and the production serum IgG in frequently relapsing EGPA patients. These events may lead to a reduction in maintenance CS intake and improve the prognosis for these patients by increasing the survival rates or decreasing the side effects of CS in patients with EGPA. It is not clear whether IVIG therapy will improve the prognosis of patients with EGPA in the long-term, because the use of IVIG may not be as popular around the world as it is in Japan and other immunosuppressive agents may be preferred therapeutic options. Much information regarding the possible mechanisms of action of IVIG has been garnered *in vitro*, but the clinical or immunologic effects of IVIG *in vivo* must be verified. It would be extremely useful clinically to determine the optimal dose level, timing of the initial dose, number of courses, and dosing interval for optimally effective IVIG therapy. Additional clinical and immunological assessment of IVIG therapy for EGPA is warranted.

ACKNOWLEDGMENTS

We thank Drs. Ikuo Saito, Ayako Horita, Hiroyuki Mitomi, and Miyako Ishiyama for their suggestions during discussions of the pathology of EGPA; Drs. Yoriko Horiguchi, Akihiko Ishibashi, Yukiko Morita, and Hideo Himeno for their suggestions during discussions of cardiac involvement; Drs. Shunsuke Suzuki, Jun Ito, Yu Sato, Takafumi Minami, and. Takahiro Tsuburai for suggestions regarding clinical manifestations; and Akemi Saito for performing the assays on the serum samples.

REFERENCES

[1] Churg J, Strauss L. Allergic granulomatosis, allergic angiitis, and periarteritis nodosa. *Am. J. Pathol.* 1951; 27:277–301.

[2] Jennette, J.C, Falk R.J. Clinical and pathological classification of ANCA associated vasculitis: what are the controversies? *Clin. Exp. Immunol.* 1995; 101:18–22.

[3] Gayraud M, Guillevin L, le Toumelin P, Cohen P, Lhote F, Casassus P, Jarrousse B; French Vasculitis Study Group. Long-term followup of polyarteritis nodosa, microscopic polyangiitis, and Churg-Strauss syndrome. *Arthritis Rheum.* 2001;:44:666–75.

[4] Guillevin L, Cohen P, Casassus P, Lhote F, Jarrousse B, Casassus P. Churg-Strauss syndrome. Clinical study and long-term follow-up of 96 patients. *Medicine.* 1999; 78:26–37.

[5] Lane SE, Watts RA, Shepstone L, Scott DG. Primary systemic vasculitis: clinical features and mortality. *Q J. Med.* 2005; 98:97–111.

[6] Chumbley L, Harrison E, DeRemee R. Allergic granulomatosis and angiitis (Churg-Strauss syndrome). *Mayo Clin. Proc.* 1977; 52:477–84.

[7] Guillevin L, Lhote F, Gayraud M, Cohen P, Jarrousse B, Lortholary O, Thibult N, Casassus P. Prognostic factors in polyarteritis nodosa and Churg-Strauss syndrome: a prospective study in 342 patients. *Medicine (Baltimore).* 1996; 75:17–28.

[8] Guillevin L, Pagnoux C, Seror R, Mahr A, Mouthon L, Toumelin P. The five-factor score revisited. Assessment of prognosis of systemic necrotizing vasculitides based on the French Vasculitis Study Group (FVSG) Cohort. *Medicine.* 2011; 90:19–27.

[9] Pagnoux C, Mahr A, Cohen P, Guillevin L. Presentation and outcome of gastrointestinal involvement in systemic necrotizing vasculitis. *Medicine.* 2005; 84:115–28.

[10] Mukhtyar C, Flossmann O, Hellmich B, Bacon P, Cid M, Cohen-Tervaert JW, Gross WL, Guillevin L, Jayne D, Mahr A, et al. European Vasculitis Study Group (EUVAS). Outcomes from studies of antineutrophil cytoplasm antibody associated vasculitis: a systemic review by the European League Against Rheumatism systemic vasculitis task force. *Ann. Rheum Dis.* 2008;67:1004–10.

[11] Pavone L, Grasselli C, Chierici E, Maggiore U, Garini G, Ronda N, Manganelli P, Pesci A, Rioda WT, Tumiati B, et al; Secondary and Primar Vasculitides (Se.Pri.Va) Study Group. Outcome and prognostic factors during the course of primary small-vessel vasculitides. *J. Rheumatol.* 2006; 33:1299–306.

[12] Ribi C, Cohen P, Pagnoux C, Mahr A, Arène JP, Lauque D, Puéchal X, Letellier P, Delaval P, Cordier JF, Guillevin L; French Vasculitis Study Group. Treatment of Churg-Strauss syndrome without poor-prognosis factors. *Arthritis Rheum.* 2008; 58:586–94.

[13] Gatenby PA, Lucas RM, Engelsen O, Ponsonby AL, Clements M. Antineutrophil cytoplasmic antibody-associated vasculitis: could geographic pattern be explained by ambient ultraviolet radiation? *Arthritis Rheum* 2009; 61: 1417-24.

[14] Mohammad AJ, Jacobsson LT, Mahr AD Sturfelt G, Segelmark M. Prevalence of Wegener's granulomatosis, microscopic polyangiitis, polyarteritis nodosa and Churg-Strauss Syndrome within a defined population in southern Sweden. *Rheumatology (Oxford)* 2007; 46: 1329-37.

[15] Mahr A, Guillevin L, Poissonnet M, Ayme S. Prevalence of polyarteritis nodosa, microscopic polyangiitis, Wegener's granulomatosis, and Churg-Strauss Syndrome in a French urban multiethnic population in 2000: a capture-recapture estimate. *Arthritis Rheum* 2004; 51: 92-9.

[16] Sinico RA, Bottero P. Churg-Strauss angiitis. *Best Pract. Res. Clin. Rheumatol.* 2009; 23:355-66.

[17] Kahn JE, Bletry O, Guillevin L. Hypereosinophilic syndromes. *Best Pract Res. Clin. Rheumatol.* 2008; 22: 863-82.

[18] Tsurikisawa N, Saito H, Oshikata C, Tsuburai T, Akiyama K. The etiology, mechanisms, and treatment of Churg-Strauss syndrome The etiology, pathogenesis and pathology of vasculitis. *InTech.* 2011 pp235-254.

[19] Pagnoux C, Guillevin L. Churg-Strauss Syndrome: evidence for disease subtypes? *Curr. Opin. Rheumatol.* 2010; 2:429-43.
[20] Radice A, Sinico RA. Antineutrophil cytoplasmic antibodies (ANCA). *Autoimmunity.* 2005; 38:93-103.
[21] Ozaki S. ANCA-associated vasculitis: diagnostic and therapeutic strategy. *Allergol Int.* 2007; 56:87-96.
[22] Keogh KA, Specks U. Churg-Strauss Syndrome: clinical presentation, antineutrophil cytoplasmic antibodies, and leukotriene receptor antagonists. *Am. J. Med.* 2003; 115: 632-8.
[23] Sinico RA, Di Toma L, Maggiore U, Bottero P, Radice A, Tosoni C, Gregorini G, Monti S, Frassi M, Vecchio F, et al. Prevalence and clinical significance of antineutrophil cytoplasmic antibodies in Churg-Strauss syndrome. *Arthritis Rheum* 2005; 52: 2926-35.
[24] Kallenberg CG. Churg-Strauss Syndrome: just one disease entity? *Arthritis Rheum* 2005; 52: 2589-93.
[25] Lhote F, Guillevin L. Polyarteritis nodosa, microscopic polyangiitis, and Churg – Strauss syndrome. Clinical aspects and treatment. *Rheum Dis Clin. North Am.* 1995; 21: 911-47.
[26] Tsurikisawa N, Tsuburai T, Saito H, Morita S, Horiguchi Y, Mitomi H, Akiyama K. A retrospective study of bronchial hyperresponsiveness in asthmatic patients prior to the onset of Churg-Strauss Syndrome. *Allergy Asthma Proc.* 2007; 28:336-43.
[27] Steinfeld S, Golstein M, De Vuyst P. Chronic eosinophilic pneumonia (CEP) as a presenting feature of Churg-Strauss syndrome (CSS). *Eur. Respir J.* 1994; 7: 2098.
[28] Marchand E, Cordier JF. Idiopathic chronic eosinophilic pneumonia. Semin Respir Crit Care Med 2006; 27:134–41.
[29] Cottin V, Cordier JF. Eosinophilic pneumonias. *Allergy* 2005; 60:841–57.
[30] Albera C, Ghio P, Solidoro P, Mabritto I, Marchetti L, Pozzi E. Activated and memory alveolar T-lymphocytes in idiopathic eosinophilic pneumonia. *Eur. Respir J.* 1995; 8:1281–5.
[31] Tsurikisawa N, Saito H, Tsuburai T, Oshikata C, Ono E, Mitomi H, Akiyama K. Differences in regulatory T cells between Churg-Strauss syndrome and chronic eosinophilic pneumonia with asthma. *J. Allergy Clin. Immunol.* 2008; 122:610–6.
[32] Sakaguchi S. Regulatory T cells: key controllers of immunologic self-tolerance. *Cell.* 2000; 101:455–8.

[33] Levings MK, Sangregorio R, Galbiati F, Squadrone S, de Waal Malefyt R, Roncarolo MG. IFN-alpha and IL-10 induce the differentiation of human type 1 T regulatory cells. *J. Immunol.* 2001; 166:5530–42.

[34] Zheng SG, Wang JH, Stohl W, Kim KS, Gray JD, Horwitz DA. TGF-beta requires CTLA-4 early after T cell activation to induce FoxP3 and generate adaptive CD4+CD25+ regulatory cells. *J. Immunol.* 2006; 176:3321–9.

[35] Valencia X, Yarboro C, Illei G, Lipsky PE. Deficient $CD4^{+}$CD25high T regulatory cell function in patients with active systemic lupus erythematosus. *J. Immunol.* 2007;178:2579–88.

[36] van Amelsfort JM, van Roon JA, Noordegraaf M, Jacobs KM, Bijlsma JW, Lafeber FP, Taams LS. Proinflammatory mediator-induced reversal of $CD4^{+}CD25^{+}$ regulatory T cell-mediated suppression in rheumatoid arthritis. *Arthritis Rheum* 2007; 56:732–42.

[37] Gottenberg JE, Lavie F, Abbed K, Gasnault J, Le Nevot E, Delfraissy JF, Taoufik Y, Mariette X. $CD4^{+}$CD25high regulatory T cells are not impaired in patients with primary Sjogren's syndrome. *J. Autoimmun* 2005; 24: 235-42.

[38] Abdulahad WH, Stegeman CA, van der Geld YM, Doornbos-van der Meer B, Limburg PC, Kallenberg CG. Functional defect of circulating regulatory $CD4^{+}$ T cells in patients with Wegener's granulomatosis in remission. *Arthritis Rheum.* 2007; 56: 2080-91.

[39] Karagiannidis C, Akdis M, Holopainen P, Woolley NJ, Hense G, Rückert B, Mantel PY, Menz G, Akdis CA, Blaser K, Schmidt-Weber CB. Glucocorticoids upregulate FOXP3 expression and regulatory T cells in asthma. *J. Allergy Clin. Immunol.* 2004; 114:1425–33.

[40] Xystrakis E, Kusumakar S, Boswell S, Peek E, Urry Z, Richards DF, Adikibi T, Pridgeon C, Dallman M, Loke TK, et al. Reversing the defective induction of IL-10-secreting regulatory T cells in glucocorticoid-resistant asthma patients. *J. Clin. Invest* 2006; 116:146–55.

[41] Saito H, Tsurikisawa N, Tsuburai T, Akiyama K. Involvement of regulatory T cells in the pathogenesis of Churg-Strauss syndrome. *Int. Arch. Allergy Immunol* 2008; 146: 73-6.

[42] Nembrini C, Maeskand BJ, Kopf M. IL-17-producing T cells in lung immunity and inflammation. *J. Allergy Clin. Immunol.* 2009; 123:986-94.

[43] Zhou L, Lopes JE, Chong MM, Ivanov II, Min R, Victora GD, Shen Y, Du J, Rubtsov YP, Rudensky AY, et al. TGF-beta-induced Foxp3

inhibits T(H)17 cell differentiation by antagonizing RORgammat function. *Nature* 2008;453:236-40.

[44] Yang XO, Nurieva R, Martinez GJ, Kang HS, Chung Y, Pappu BP, Shah B, Chang SH, Schluns KS, Watowich SS, et al. Molecular antagonism and plasticity of regulatory and inflammatory T cell programs. *Immunity*. 2008; 29:44-56.

[45] Arnaud L, Haroche J, Mathian A, Gorochov G, Amoura Z. Pathogenesis of Takayasu's arteritis: a 2011 update. *Autoimmun Rev*. 2011;11:61-7.

[46] Terrier B, Geri G, Chaara W, Allenbach Y, Rosenzwajg M, Costedoat-Chalumeau N, Fouret P, Musset L, Benveniste O, Six A, et al. Interleukin-21 modulates Th1 and Th17 responses in giant cell arteritis. *Arthritis Rheum*. 2012;64:2001-11.

[47] Jen HY, Chuang YH, Lin SC, Chiang BL, Yang YH. Increased serum interleukin-17 and peripheral Th17 cells in children with acute Henoch-Schönlein purpura. *Pediatr Allergy Immunol*. 2011;22:862-8.

[48] Kallenberg CG. Pathogenesis of ANCA-associated vasculitis, an update. *Clin. Rev. Allergy Immunol*. 2011;41:224-31.

[49] Nogueira E, Hamour S, Sawant D, Henderson S, Mansfield N, Chavele KM, Pusey CD, Salama AD. Serum IL-17 and IL-23 levels and autoantigen-specific Th17 cells are elevated in patients with ANCA-associated vasculitis. *Nephrol. Dial Transplant* 2010;25:2209-17.

[50] Abdulahad WH, Stegeman CA, Limburg PC, Kallenberg CG. Skewed distribution of Th17 lymphocytes in patients with Wegener's granulomatosis in remission. *Arthritis Rheum*. 2008;58:2196-205.

[51] Jakiela B, Sanak M, Szczeklik W, Sokolowska B, Plutecka H, Mastalerz L, Musial J, Szczeklik A. Both Th2 and Th17 responses are involved in the pathogenesis of Churg-Strauss syndrome. *Clin. Exp. Rheumatol*. 2011;29:S23-34.

[52] Saito H, Tsurikisawa N, Tsuburai T, Oshikata C, Akiyama K. Cytokine production profile of $CD4^+$ T cells from patients with active Churg-Strauss syndrome tends toward Th17. *Int. Arch. Allergy Immunol*. 2009;149 Suppl 1:61-5.

[53] Terrier B, Bièche I, Maisonobe T, Laurendeau I, Rosenzwajg M, Kahn JE, Diemert MC, Musset L, Vidaud M, Sène D, et al. Interleukin-25: a cytokine linking eosinophils and adaptive immunity in Churg-Strauss syndrome. *Blood*. 2010;116:4523-31.

[54] Saito H, Tsurikisawa N, Tsuburai T, Oshikata C, Akiyama K. The proportion of regulatory T cells in the peripheral blood reflects the

relapse or remission status of patients with Churg-Strauss syndrome. *Int Arch. Allergy Immunol.* 2011; 155; 46-52.
[55] Stumhofer JS, Laurence A, Wilson EH, Huang E, Tato CM, Johnson LM, Villarino AV, Huang Q, Yoshimura A, Sehy D, et al. Interleukin 27 negatively regulates the development of interleukin 17-producing T helper cells during chronic inflammation of the central nervous system. *Nat. Immunol.* 2006; 7:937-45.
[56] Saito H, Tsurikisawa N, Oshikata C, Tsuburai T, Akiyama K. Increased interleukin-27 production by antigen-presenting cells promotes regulatory T cell differentiation and contributes to inducing a remission in patients with eosinophilic granulomatosis with polyangiitis. *Int. Arch. Allergy Immunol.* 2013;161 Suppl 2:66-74.
[57] Tsurikisawa N, Saito H, Oshikata C, Tsuburai T, Akiyama K. Decreases in the numbers of peripheral blood regulatory T cells, and increases in the levels of memory and activated B cells, in patients with active eosinophilic granulomatosis and polyangiitis. *J. Clin. Immunol.* 2013; 33: 965-76.
[58] Vaglio A, Buzio C, Zwerina J. Eosinophilic granulomatosis with polyangiitis (Churg-Straus): State of the art. *Allergy* 2013; 68:261-73.
[59] Abril A, Calamia KT, Cohen MD. The Churg Strauss syndrome (allergic granulomatous angiitis): review and update. *Semin. Arthritis Rheum* 2003; 33: 106-14.
[60] Hattori N, Ichimura M, Nagamatsu M, Li M, Yamamoto K, Kumazawa K, Mitsuma T, Sobue G. Clinicopathological features of Churg-Strauss syndrome-associated neuropathy. *Brain* 1999; 122, 427-39.
[61] Sehgal M, Swanson JW, DeRemee RA, Colby TV. Neurological manifestations of Churg-Strauss syndrome. *Mayo Clin. Proc.* 1995; 70: 337-341.
[62] Renaldini E, Spandrio S, Cerudelli A, Affatato A, Balestrieri GP. Cardiac involvement in Churg-Strauss syndrome: a follow-up of three cases. *Eur. Heart J.* 1993; 14: 1712-1716.
[63] Rees JR, Burgess P. An abdominal presentation of Churg-strauss syndrome. *Case Rep. Med.* 2010; Article ID 290654.
[64] Hashida G, Kan A, Inoue S, Abe K. Rehabilitation method for churg-strauss syndrome from early stage: considering functional prognosis of mononeuritis multiplex. *No To Shinkei.* 2006; 58:425-9.
[65] Tsurikisawa N, Taniguchi M, Suzuki S, Akiyama K. Effects of a nitro compound patch on neuropathy in Churg-Strauss syndrome. *Allergy* 2003; 58:686-7.

[66] Jayne DRW, Davies MJ, Fox CJV, Black CM, Lockwood CM. Treatment of systemic vasculitis with pooled intravenous immunoglobulin. *Lancet* 1991; 337: 1137-1139.

[67] Lockwood CM. New treatment strategies for systemic vasculitis: the role of intravenous immunoglobulin therapy. *Clin. Exp. Imunol.* 1996; 104: 77-82.

[68] Richter C, Schnabel A, Csernok E, De Groot K, Reinhold-Keller E, Gross WL. Treatment of anti-neutrophil cytoplasmic antibody (ANCA)-associated systemic vasculitis with high-dose intravenous immunoglobulin. *Clin. Exp. Immunol.* 1995; 101:2-7.

[69] Martinez V, Cohen P, Pagnoux C, Vinzio S, Mahr A, Mouthon L, Sailler L, Delaunay C, Sadoun A, Guillevin L; French Vasculitis Study Group. Intravenous immunoglobulins for relapses of systemic vasculitides associated with antineutrophil cytoplasmic autoantibodies: results of a multicenter, prospective, open-label study of twenty-two patients. *Arthritis Rheum.* 2008; 58:308-17.

[70] Hamilos DL, Christensen J. Treatment of Churg-Strauss syndrome with high-dose intravenous immunoglobulin. *J. Allergy Clin. Immunol* 1991; 88: 823-824.

[71] Armentia A, Fernández A, Sánchez P, de la Fuente R, Sanchís E, Méndez J, Parra I, Puyo M. Asthma and vasculitis. Response to intravenous immunoglobulins. *Allergol. Immunopathol. (Madr)* 1993 ; 21: 47-52.

[72] Levy Y, George J, Fabbrizzi F, Rotman P, Paz Y, Shoenfeld Y. Marked improvement of Churg-Strauss vasculitis with intravenous gammaglobulins. *South Med. J.* 1999; 92: 412-414.

[73] Tsurikisawa N, Taniguchi T, Saito H, Himeno H, Ishibashi A, Suzuki S, Akiyama K. Treatment of Churg-Strauss syndrome with high-dose intravenous immunoglobulin. *Ann. Allerg Asthma Immunol.* 2004; 92:80–7.

[74] Guillevin L, Pagnoux C. When should immunosuppressants be prescribed to treat systemic vasculitides? *Internal Med.* 2003; 42: 313–317.

[75] Kazatchkine MD, Kaveri SV. Immunomoduration of autoimmune and inflammatory disease with intravenous immune globulin. *N. Engl. J. Med.* 2001; 345: 747-55.

[76] Mackay, Ian R; Rosen, Fred S; Kazatchkine, Michel D; Kaveri, Srini V. Immunomodulation of autoimmune and inflammatory diseases with intravenous immune globulin. *New Eng. J. Med.* 2001; 345: 747-755.

[77] Maddur MS, Othy S, Hegde P, Vani J, Lacroix-Desmazes S, Bayry J, Kaveri SV. Immunomodulation by intravenous immunoglobulin: role of regulatory T cells. *J. Clin. Immunol.* 2010; 30(Suppl 1): S4-S8.

[78] Cousens LP, Najafian N, Mingozzi F, Elyaman W, Mazer B, Moise L, Messitt TJ, Su Y, Sayegh M, High K, et al. In vitro and in vivo studies of IgG-derived Treg epitopes (Tregitopes): a promising new tool for tolerance induction and treatment of autoimmunity. *J. Clin. Immunol.* 2013;33 Suppl 1:S43-9.

[79] Kessel A, Ammuri H, Peri R, Pavlotzky ER, Blank M, Shoenfeld Y, Toubi E. Intravenous immunoglobulin therapy affects T regulatory cells by increasing their suppressive function. *J. Immunol.* 2007;179:5571–5575.

[80] De Groot AS, Moise L, MucMurry JA, Wambre E, Van Overtvelt L, Moingeon P, Scott DW, Martin W. Activation of natural regulatory T cells by IgG Fc-derived peptide “Tergitopes”. *Blood* 2008;112:3303–3311.

[81] Nimmerjahn F, Ravetch JV. Anti-inflammatory actions of intravenous immunogloblin. *Annu Rev. Immunol.* 2008;26:513–533.

[82] Tha-In T, Metselaar HJ, Bushell AR, Kwekkeboom J, Wood KJ. Intravenous immunoglobulins promote skin allograft acceptance by triggering functional activation of $CD4^{+}Foxp3^{+}$ T cells. *Transplantation* 2010;89:1446–1455.

[83] Anthony RM, Kobayashi T, Wermeling F, Ravetch JV. Intravenous gammaglobulin suppresses inflammation through a novel T(H)2 pathway. *Nature.*2011;475:110-3.

[84] Maddur MS, Vani J, Hegde P, Lacroix-Desmazes S, Kaveri SV, Bayry J. Inhibition of differentiation, amplification, and function of human TH17 cells by intravenous immunoglobulin. *J. Allergy Clin. Immunol.* 2011;127:823-30.

[85] Séïté JF, Cornec D, Renaudineau Y, Youinou P, Mageed RA, Hillion S. IVIg modulates BCR signaling through CD22 and promotes apoptosis in mature human B lymphocytes. *Blood.* 2010; 116:1698-704.

[86] Tsurikisawa N, Saito H, Oshikata C, Tsuburai T, Akiyama K. High-dose intravenous immunoglobulin treatment increases regulatory T cells in patients with eosinophilic granulomatosis with polyangiitis. *J. Rheumatol.* 2012; 39:1019–1025.

[87] Danieli MG, Cappelli M, Malcangi G, Logullo F, Salvi A, Danieli G. Long term effectiveness of intravenous immunoglobulin in Churg–Strauss syndrome. *Ann. Rheum Dis.* 2004; 63:1649–1654.

[88] von Gunten S, Vogel M, Schaub A, Stadler BM, Miescher S, Crocker PR, Simon HU. Intravenous immunoglobulin preparations contain anti-Siglec-8 autoantibodies. *J. Allergy Clin. Immunol.* 2007; 119:1005-11.

[89] Tsurikisawa N, Saito H, Oshikata C, Tsuburai T, Akiyama K. High-dose intravenous immunoglobulin therapy for eosinophilic granulomatosis with polyangiitis. 2014 submitted.

[90] Moosig F, Bremer JP, Hellmich B, Holle JU, Holl-Ulrich K, Laudien M, Matthis C, Metzler C, Nölle B, Richardt G, Gross WL. A vasculitis centre based management strategy leads to improved outcome in eosinophilic granulomatosis and polyangiitis (Churg-Strauss, EGPA): monocentric experiences in 150 patients. *Ann. Rheum. Dis.* 2013; 72:1011-7.

[91] Horiguchi Y, Morita Y, Tsurikisawa N, Akiyama K. 123I-MIBG imaging detects cardiac involvement and predicts cardiac events in Churg-Strauss syndrome. *Eur. J. Nucl. Med. Mol. Imaging* 2011; 38: 221-9.

In: Plasmapheresis and Intravenous … ISBN: 978-1-63117-916-7
Editor: Rossana Allegro

Chapter 6

THERAPY WITH IMMUNOGLOBULIN IN PATIENTS WITH ACUTE MYOCARDITIS

Chiharu Kishimoto*
Dpartment of Cardiovascular Medicine, Graduate School of Medicine,
Kyoto University, Japan

ABSTRACT

Intravenous immunoglobulin (IVIG) therapy has been used to treat several autoimmune or inflammatory diseases. We conducted a clinical trial of immunoglobulin therapy for acute myocarditis. The study consisted of the following: a comparison of prognosis between the patients treated with and those not treated with IVIG in multi-center study. 15 patients were treated with IVIG (1-2g/kg, over 2 days), whereas 26 were untreated. There was a statistically significant difference between the survival curves of the patients treated with IVIG (20.0%, 3/15) and the survival curves of those not treated with IVIG (34.6%, 9/26). There was no significant difference between the IVIG-treated and untreated groups in terms of clinical parameters of acute and chronic phases. Therefore, therapy with IVIG seems to be a promising treatment for acute myocarditis given that it improves the clinical course.

---

* Address for correspondence: Chiharu Kishimoto, MD, PhD, Department of Cardiovascular Medicine, Graduate School of Medicine, Kyoto University, 54 Kawara-cho, Shogoin, Sakyo-ku, Kyoto 606-8507, Japan, Tel: (81) 075-751-3197 Fax: (81) 075-751-4281, E-mail: kkishi@kuhp.kyoto-u.ac.jp.

Keywords: Acute myocarditis; IVIG; Cytokine; Fc receptors

INTRODUCTION

Clinical manifestations of myocarditis generally consist of electrocardiographic abnormalities, enzymatic disorders, and the occurrence of heart failure and sudden death [1-3]. However, limited success has been reported for the treatments of inflammatory myocardial diseases such as corticosteroid and cytotoxic drugs [4-7]. Furthermore, the need for continuing treatment exposed the patient to the risk of long-term immunosuppressive therapy.

Myocarditis, especially viral myocarditis, is considered to be a cause of dilated cardiomyopathy [8, 9]. Immune or autoimmune mechanisms may be involved in the pathogenesis of myocarditis and subsequent cardiomyopathy. It was reported that T cells play a role in the development of myocarditis [8]; the severity of myocarditis is regulated not by B cells but by T cells.

Intravenous immunoglobulin (IVIG) therapy has been used to treat several autoimmune conditions, including Kawasaki disease, idiopathic thrombocytopenic purpura, and systemic vasculitis [10, 11], but its mechanisms of action is unclear, and may vary among conditions. Previous studies [10, 11] have revealed several mechanisms; neutralization of pathogens, attenuation of complement-mediated tissue damage, anti-inflammatory activity mediated through the inhibitory Fc receptor, and acceleration of pathogenic immunoglobulin catabolism. We have previously shown that immunoglobulin therapy suppresses experimental myocarditis through its antiviral effects as well as by reducing inflammatory cytokines [12, 13]. Here, we report the results of a multi-center trial of IVIG therapy for acute myocarditis along with a substudy in which inflammatory cytokines and peripheral leukocyte profiles were analyzed.

METHODS

Study Protocol

Patients were recruited from cardiology departments of the institutes. The primary inclusion criteria were a left ventricular ejection fraction (LVEF) of

≤0.40 and no more than 6 months of cardiac symptoms at the time of randomization. Patients were eligible if they presented with acute cardiac failure or arrhythmia and with a history of a recent flu-like illness with electrocardiographic abnormalities [1-3]. Exclusion criteria were diabetes, thyroid disease, renal disease, uncontrolled hypertension (systolic blood pressure>140mmHg and diastolic blood pressure>90mmHg), valvular heart disease or previous history of documented ischemic heart disease [1-3].

The study consisted of two parts. One was a multi-center comparison of survival and prognosis between the patients treated with IVIG and those who were not treated with IVIG (non-IVIG), and the other was an analysis of inflammatory cytokines and blood cell profiles that was conducted in a substudy. The substudy was part of the multi-center study.

Written informed consent was obtained from all of the study patients, and the study protocol was approved by the ethics committee of the institutes.

The study included 41 patients (27 male, 14 female; aged 19-80 years). After obtaining informed consent, the patients were randomly divided into two groups. Fifteen patients were treated with high-dose IVIG (1-2g/kg, over 2 days), and 26 were untreated and served as a control arm. The histological diagnosis of myocarditis was made based on the Dallas criteria [14]. The mean duration of disease before IVIG was 2.2 months (range; 1-6 months). Patients with so-called eosinophilic myocarditis were excluded from the study [15, 16]. Patients with dilated cardiomyopathy were eligible for this study if they presented with signs or symptoms of congestive heart failure of <6 months duration and a left ventricular ejection fraction (LVEF) of ≤40%. Twenty patients (48.8%) underwent pretreatment catheterization (including coronary arteriography) with an endomyocardial biopsy. Routine pathological evaluations were performed using obtained specimens; immunohistochemistry and in situ hybridization for myocardial viruses were performed in some cases.

After obtaining baseline LVEF and laboratory data, IVIG was administered over a period of 48 hours. The patients received a total dose of 1-2 g/kg. Immunoglobulin preparations used in this study were all intact types (Fc portion; Venilon, Polyglobin-N, and Venoglobulin-IH). All patients received continuous cardiac monitoring during IVIG therapy.

Clinical characteristics of the patients, the ejection fraction of the left ventricle as assessed by echocardiography, the presence or absence of a circulatory assist device, and the degree of recovery were analyzed. The difference between acute stage and recovery stage was determined by symptoms and clinical parameters as well as courses. Incomplete recovery following the application of therapy was defined as the presence of symptoms with evidence of disease activity, and complete recovery was defined as the absence of symptoms.

Statistical Analyses

Continuous values are represented as mean±SD. Categorical values are represented as a number or percentage. Statistical analysis was performed with the unpaired *t* test for continuous variables, and Fisher's exact test or χ^2 test as appropriate for categorical variables. Survival curves were analyzed by Kaplan-Meier methods. A value of $P<0.05$ was considered statistically significant.

RESULTS

There was a statistically significant difference ($P<0.01$) between the survival curves of the patients treated with IVIG and the survival curves of those who were not treated with IVIG. Namely, there was a tendency for a lower mortality rate in the IVIG treated group (20.0%, 3/15) compared with the untreated group (34.6 %, 9/26). The cause of death was myocardial pump failure in both groups. There was no significant difference between IVIG-treated and untreated groups in terms of the parameters of acute- as well as chronic-phase ejection fractions of the left ventricle, the percentages of patients with a circulatory assist device, or prognosis (death and complete recovery) of the disease.

No significant viruses detected by the paired assay in the sera of all patients.

The first histological examinations were performed 14.1±6.0 days (range 3-38 days) from the onset of myocarditis, and these demonstrated lymphocytic myocarditis in 16 (39.0%, 16/41) patients in the study groups among those, 1 (2.4%) was affected with giant cells myocarditis. These patients showed infiltration of inflammatory cells into the myocardium with necrosis or degeneration of cardiomyocytes, and the findings met the criterion for active myocarditis according to the Dallas criteria [14]. Five (12.2%) patients were diagnosed as having borderline myocarditis [14]. Fifteen (36.6%) patients were diagnosed as having acute dilated cardiomyopathy.

All patients were hospitalized with New York Heart Association (NYHA) class III or IV symptoms. Eleven of 15 patients (73.3%) in IVIG group and 23 out of 26 patients (88.5%) in the non-IVIG group received IABP or PCPS support during the hospitalization. All patients demonstrated an improvement in LVEF; the mean LVEF for IVIG group improved from 17.2 ±9.0% to 41.4±13.3%, and that for the non-IVIG group from 29.8 ±11.5% to 56.9 ±17.0%.

All patients tolerated the therapy without serious complications or side effects, and were followed up for a median of 3.5 months after therapy (range, 3-54 months).

DISCUSSION

The therapeutic efficacy of immunoglobulin in inflammatory and autoimmune diseases has been reported [10, 11, 17]. The mechanisms responsible for the efficacy of this treatment are, however, unknown. The successful treatment of idiopathic thrombocytopenic purpura with immunoglobulin appears to result from the blockade of Fc receptors. One possible mechanism of action of IVIG in Kawasaki disease is the neutralization of a microbial toxin by immunoglobulin [18], which binds nonspecifically to certain variable regions of the T-cell- antigen receptor.

Drucker et al. [18] reported potential benefits of IVIG, in the treatment of children with recent-onset of myocarditis. Subsequently, McNamara et al. [19] reported the successful treatment of adult patients with acute cardiomyopathy by IVIG, which was associated with improved recovery of left ventricular function. Most recently, some investigators reported that IVIG may be useful for patients with chronic cardiomyopathy of left ventricular dysfunction [20-24]. In addition, Gullest et al. [24] reported that IVIG was effective for patients with heart failure, and acted by modulating cytokine balance. We have previously demonstrated that immunoglobulin therapy suppressed murine myocarditis [12, 13].

In the present study, the multi-center data indicated that the use of IVIG was associated with the amelioration of the course of the disease, an increase in left ventricular performance after the therapy, and a tendency for a lower mortality rate.

It has been suggested that cytokines play an important role in the development of inflammatory myocardial disease. For example, TNF-α inhibits the response of isolated myocytes toβ-adrenergic stimuli [25]. Furthermore, TNF and interferon-γ are important mediator in the pathogenesis of myocardial inflammation in experimental myocarditis. The reduction of cytokines by immunoglobulin administration was reported as a possible therapeutic mechanism in some inflammatory diseases [17], because immunoglobulin itself contains antibodies against various cytokines [10, 11]. Recently, suppression of cytokine-dependent T-cell proliferation by immunoglobulin treatment was demonstrated in in vitro experiments and in inflammatory disorders [11]. Most recently, anti-inflammatory activity of immunoglobulin via Fc portion was demonstrated [24, 25], and the anti-inflammatory mechanisms of IVIG may be due to the inhibitory Fc receptor, Fcγ receptor IIB [26, 27]. These immunomodulatory effects of immunoglobulin via the inhibitory receptor Fcγ receptor IIB may be significant in terms of therapeutic actions in immune-mediated diseases. Most recently, it was reported that IVIG treatment ameliorated myocardial diseases to some extent in an Intervention in Myocarditis and Acute Cardiomyopathy with Immune Globulin (IMAC) trial of human myocarditis [28] and the other trial [29, 30].

Comparing the clinical characteristics of this study with those of other studies (e.g., IMAC group [28] and Fuse et al. [31]), very high prevalences of IABP and mechanical support were noted, which may account for the relatively good prognoses of the present study groups.

In conclusion, IVIG seems to be a promising agent in the treatment of acute myocarditis. The current study may shed light on the key mechanism of action of IVIG for clinical myocarditis, irrespective of the small population studied.

ACKNOWLEDGEMENTS

This study was supported in part by research grants from the Japanese Ministry of Education, Science, and Culture (18590772 and 23591040), Shimizu Immunology Foundation, All Coffee Association, The Univers Foundation, and Cardiovascular Research Foundation.

REFERENCES

[1] Kumar, K.; Guirgis, M.; Zieroth, S.; Lo, E.; Menkis, A.H.; Arora, R.C.; Freed, D.H. (2011). Influenza myocarditis and myositis: case presentation and review of the literature. *Can J Cardiol*, 27, 514-522.

[2] Schultheiss, H.P.; Kühl, U.; Cooper, L.T. (2011). The management of myocarditis. *Eur Heart J*, 32, 2616-2625.

[3] Kishimoto, C. (2011). Serial electrocardiographic changes in fulminant myocarditis. *Circ J,* 75, 2511.

[4] Mason, J.W.; O'Connel, J.B.; Herskowitz, A.; Rose, N.R.; McManus, B.M.; Billingham, M.E.; Moon, T.E. (1995). A clinical trial of immunosuppressive therapy for myocarditis. *N Engl J Med*, 333, 269-275.

[5] Wojnicz, R.; Nowalany-Kozielska, E.; Wojciechowska, C.; Glanowska, G.; Wilczewski, P.; Niklewski, T.; Zembala, M.; Polonski, L.; Rozek, M.M.; Wodniecki, J. (2001). Randomized, placebo-controlled study for immunosuppressive treatment of inflammatory dilated cardiomyopathy. Two-year follow-up results. *Circulation*, 104, 39-45.

[6] Hirano, E.; Shimada, K.; Komiyama, T.; Fujita, M.; Kishimoto, C. (2013). Erythromycin treatment suppresses myocardial injury in autoimmune myocarditis in rats via suppression of superoxide production. *Int J Cardiol,* 167, 2228-2233.

[7] Kishimoto, C.; Nimata, M.; Okabe, T.A.; Shioji, K. (2013). Immunoglobulin treatment ameliorates myocardial injury in experimental autoimmune myocarditis associated with suppression of reactive oxygen species. *Int J Cardiol*, 167, 140-145.

[8] Kawai, C. (1999). From myocarditis to cardiomyopathy. Mechanisms of inflammation and cell death. *Circulation*, 99, 1091-1100.

[9] Richardson, P.; McKenna, W.; Bristow, M.; Maisch, B.; Mautner, B.; O'Connell, J.; Olsen, E.; Thiene, G.; Goodwin, J.; Gyarfas, I.; Martin, I.; Nordet, P. (1996). Report of the 1995 World Health Organization/International Society of Federation of Cardiology. Task force on the definition and classification of cardiomyopathies. *Circulation*, 93, 841-842.

[10] Wolf, H.M.; Eibl, M.M. (1996). Immunodulatory effect of immunoglobulins. *Clin Exp Rheum*, 14 (Suppl 15), S17-25.

[11] Rosen, F.S. (1993). Putative mechanisms of the effect of intravenous γ-globulin. *Clin Immunol Immunopathol*, 67, S41-43.

[12] Takada, H.; Kishimoto, C.; Hiraoka, Y. (1995). Therapy with immunoglobulin suppresses myocarditis in a murine coxsackievirus B3 model: antiviral and anti-inflammatory effects. *Circulation*, 92, 1604-1611.

[13] Kishimoto, C.; Takamatsu, N.; Kawamata, H.; Shinohara, H.; Ochiai, H. (2000). Immunoglobulin treatment ameliorates murine myocarditis associated with reduction of neurohumoral activity and improvement of extracellular matrix change. *J Am Coll Cardiol*, 36, 1979-1984.

[14] Aretz, H.T.; Billingham, M.E.; Edwards, W.D.; Factor, S.M.; Fenoglio, J.T.; Fenoglio, J.J. Jr.; Olsen, E.G.; Schoen, F.J. (1987). Myocarditis. A histopathologic definition and classification. *Am J Cardiovasc Pathol*, 1, 3-14.

[15] Al, A.A.; Straatman, L.P.; Allard, M.F.; Ignaszewski, A.P. (2006). Eosinophilic myocarditis. Case series and review of literature. *Can J Cardiol*, 14, 1233-1237.

[16] Morimoto, S.; Kubo, N.; Hiramitsu, S.; Demura, A.; Ohtuki, M.; Kato, S.; Kato, Y.; Sugiura, A.; Miyagishima, K.; Mori, N.; Yoshida, Y.; Hishida, H.; (2003). Changes in the peripheral eosinophilic count in patients with acute eosinophilic myocarditis. *Heart Vessels*, 4, 193-196.

[17] Anthony, R.M.; Kobayashi, T.; Wermeling, F.; Ravetch, J.V. (2011). Intravenous gammagloblin suppresses inflammation through a novel T(H)2 pathway. *Nature*, 475, 110-113.

[18] Drucker, N.A.; Colan, S.D.; Lewis, A.B.; Beiser, A.S.; Wessel, D.L.; Takahashi, M.; Baker, A.L.; Perez-Atayde, A.R.; Newburger, J.W. (1994). Gamma-globulin treatment of acute myocarditis in the pediatric population. *Circulation*, 89, 252-257.

[19] McNamara, D.M.; Rosenblum, W.D.; Janosko, K.M.; Trost, M.K.; Villaneuva, F.S.; Demetris, A.J.; Murali, S.; Feldman, A.M. (1997). Intravenous immune globulin in the therapy of myocarditis and acute cardiomyopathy. *Circulation*, 95, 2476-2478.

[20] Felix, S.B.; Staudt, A.; Dörffel, W.V.; Stangl, V.; Merkel, K.; Pohl, M.; Döcke, W.D.; Morgera, S.; Neumayer, H.H.; Wernecke, K.D.; Wallukat, G.; Stangl, K.; Baumann, G. (2000). Hemodynamic effects of substitution and subsequent immunoglobulin substitution in dilated cardiomyopathy. *J Am Coll Cardiol,* 35, 1590-1598.

[21] Bozkurt, B.; Villaneuva, M.D.; Holubkov, R.; Tokarczyk, T.; Alvarez, R.J. Jr.; MacGowan, G.A.; Murali, S.; Rosenblum, W.D.; Feldman, A.M.; McNamara, D.M. (1999). Intravenous immune globulin in the therapy of peripartum cardiomyopathy. *J Am Coll Cardiol*, 34, 177-180.

[22] Damås, J.K.; Gullestad, L.; Aass, H.; Simonsen, S.; Fjeld, J.G.; Wikeby, L.; Ueland, T.; Eiken, H.G.; Frøland, S.S.; Aukrust, P. (2001). Enhanced gene expression of chemokines and their corresponding receptors in mononuclear blood cells in chronic heart failure. Modulatory effect of intravenous immunoglobulin. *J Am Coll Cardiol*, 38, 187-193.

[23] Staudt, A.; Schäper, F.; Stangl, V.; Plagemann, A.; Böhm, M.; Markel, K.; Wallukat, G.; Wernecke, K.D.; Stangl, K.; Baumann, G.; Felix, S.B. (2001). Immunological changes in dilated cardiomyopathy induced by immunoadsorption therapy and subsequent immunoglobulin substitution. *Circulation*, 103, 2681-2686.

[24] Gullestad, L.; Aass, H.; Fjeld, J.G.; Wikeby, L.; Andreassen, A.K.; Ihlen, H.; Simonsen, S.; Kjekshus, J.; Nitter-Hauge, S.; Ueland, T.; Lien, E.; Frøland, S.S.; Ankrust, P. (2001). Immunomodulating therapy with intravenous immunoglobulin in patients with chronic heart failure. *Circulation*, 103, 220-225.

[25] Geng, Y.; Hansson, G.K.; Holme, E. (1992). Interferon-γ and tumor necrosis factor synergize to induce nitric oxide production and inhibit mitochondrial respiration in vascular smooth muscle cells. *Circ Res*, 71, 1268-1276.

[26] Samuelsson, A.; Towers, T.L.; Ravetch, J.V. (2001). Anti-inflammatory activity of IVIG mediated through the inhibitory Fc receptor. *Science*, 291, 484-486.

[27] Shioji, K.; Kishimoto, C.; Sasayama, S. (2001). Fc receptor-mediated inhibitory effect of immunoglobulin therapy upon autoimmune giant cell myocarditis. Concomitant suppression of the expression of dendritic cells *Circ Res,* 89, 540-546.

[28] McNamara, D.M.; Holubkov, R.; Starling, R.C.; Dec, G.W.; Loh, E.; Torre-Amione, G.; Gass, A.; Karen, J. (2001). Controlled trial of intravenous immune globulin in recent-onset dilated cardiomyopathy. *Circulation*, 103, 2254-2259.

[29] Schimke, I.; Müller, J.; Priem, F.; Kruse, I.; Schön, B.; Stein, J.; Kunze, R.; Wallukat, G.; Hetzer, R. (2001). Decreased oxidative stress in patients with idiopathic dilated cardiomyopathy one year after immunoglobulin adsorption. *J Am Coll Cardiol*, 38, 178-183.

[30] Trucco, S.M.; Jaeggi, E.; Cuneo, B.; Moon-Grady, A.J.; Silverman, E.; Silverman, N.; Hornberger, L.K. (2011). Use of intravenous gamma globulin and corticosteroids in the treatment of maternal autoantibody-mediated cardiomyopathy. *J Am Coll Cardiol*, 57, 715-723.

[31] Fuse, K.; Kodama, M.; Okura, Y.; Ito, M.; Hirono, S.; Kato, K.; Hanawa, H.; Aizawa, Y.; (2000). Predictors of disease course in patients with acute myocarditis. *Circulation*, 102, 2829-2835.

In: Plasmapheresis and Intravenous ... ISBN: 978-1-63117-916-7
Editor: Rossana Allegro

Chapter 7

THERAPEUTIC USE OF AUTOLOGOUS PLASMA FOR THE TREATMENT OF DRY EYE DISEASE

Beau J. Fenner and Louis Tong*
Duke-NUS Graduate Medical School, Singapore
Singapore Eye Research Institute, Singapore
Singapore National Eye Centre, Singapore

ABSTRACT

Dry eye disease is a common ophthalmic condition that results from a complex interplay between tear production and the ocular surface, producing symptoms of discomfort, visual impairment, and tear film instability that can damage the ocular surface. Numerous treatment options for mild forms of dry eye disease exist, including lifestyle changes, artificial tears, tear secretagogues, and punctum plugging. More severe dry eye disease, however, is often unresponsive to conservative treatments because of the underlying damage to the ocular surface epithelium. The multitude of growth factors, cytokines, antimicrobials, and vitamins present in natural tears that normally supports the ocular surface epithelium is lacking in artificial tear solutions.

* Corresponding author: Louis Tong, MBBS, FRCS, DM, PhD. Cornea and External Eye Disease Service, Singapore National Eye Centre (SNEC) and Ocular Surface Research Group, Singapore Eye Research Institute (SERI), 11 Third Hospital Avenue Singapore 168751. Tel: +65 6227 7255, Fax: +65 6322 4599, E-mail: louis.tong.h.c@snec.com.sg.

Blood-derived serum and plasma, however, contain many of the same components as the natural tear film and have been explored over the past decade as an alternative treatment option for patients who have failed more conventional treatments. Recent clinical trials have demonstrated the benefits of serum for dry eye disease and other ocular surface disorders, with improved patient symptoms, reduced ocular surface damage and improved healing. Trials using plasma prepared by plasmapheresis have shown similar benefits, with the benefit of improved contamination control in plasmapheresis compared to standard serum preparation methods. In this chapter we discuss the current role of plasma in dry eye disease treatment, the use of plasmapheresis and related techniques for the preparation of treatment solutions, and the potential for future large-scale adoption of this method by clinicians and their patients.

Dry Eye Disease

Ophthalmologists define dry eye disease as a disease of tears and the ocular surface, producing discomfort, visual changes, and tear film instability with potential for damage to the ocular surface [1]. Recent estimates of disease prevalence indicate that it may affect up to 33% of the general population to varying degrees, with women and individuals over 60 years of age being affected more commonly [1-4]. The treatment of dry eye disease has created a substantial economic burden in industrialized nations, with recent studies indicating that the direct and indirect costs of dry eye disease likely exceed US$1000 per patient per year [5-8]. Clinically, we can approach dry eye disease by dividing the disease into either aqueous-deficiency or evaporative disease. Aqueous deficiency disease is separated into Sjögren syndrome or non-Sjögren disorders, while evaporative disease can be either intrinsic (e.g., meibomian gland dysfunction) or extrinsic (e.g., contact lens use). In addition, it is common that patients experience elements of both types of disease, resulting in a mixed dry eye disorder. A commonly employed diagnostic algorithm is shown in Figure 1. Treatment options for dry eye also take into account the severity of disease, with the 2007 International Dry Eye Workshop (DEWS) report providing four levels of severity based on symptoms, conjunctival and corneal staining, degree of meibomian gland dysfunction, tear film stability, and tear production [1]. The etiology of dry eye disease varies with disease subtype, although it is now believed that tear film hyperosmolarity and tear film instability play a crucial role in the development of disease in most individuals.

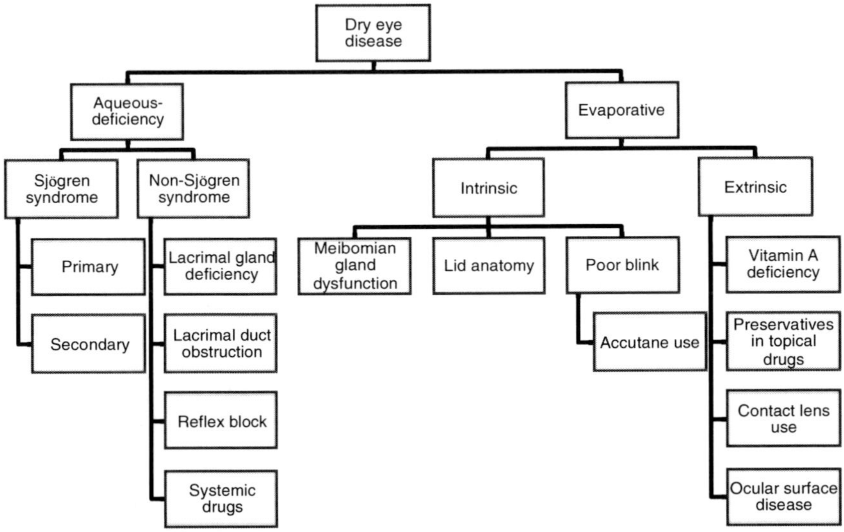

Adapted from the Dry Eye Workshop Symposium (DEWS) [1].

Figure 1. Diagnostic approach to dry eye disease.

Damage to the ocular surface epithelium by a hyperosmolar tear film results in the activation of inflammatory signaling cascades, including the NF-κB and MAP kinase pathways, that results in the production of pro-inflammatory and pro-apoptotic cytokines.

Apoptosis of goblet cells via apoptosis leads to a decline in mucin production, causing tear film instability and tear evaporation. This leads to a further increase in tear hyperosmolarity, leading to a vicious cycle of worsening ocular surface health and increased symptoms of dry eye disease.

Clinically, dry eye symptoms are typically assessed using a battery of relatively simple subjective and objective tests.

Dry eye symptoms are commonly graded with a visual analogue "faces" scale. Clinical examinations include a Schirmer test to quantify tear volume, tear break-up time (TBUT) to assess tear film stability, corneal fluorescein staining for corneal damage, and evaluation of the lid margins for meibomian gland function.

There remains significant debate within the ophthalmology community about how best to score dry eye disease, although the DEWS report mentioned above provides a framework for clinicians to approach this problem.

Current Treatment Modalities for Dry Eye Disease

Successful management of dry eye disease should reduce the symptoms and signs of inflammation, and restore a normal ocular surface. Initial efforts to manage dry eye usually involve modifying or eliminating any environment-tal factors that may be causing or contributing to the disease, while associated medical conditions such as Sjögren syndrome are managed in consultation with a specialist in the relevant area. Counseling patients on the importance of proper lid hygiene is also important and is often sufficient to improve dry eye symptoms when meibomian gland dysfunction and posterior blepharitis are the major culprits in the disease. Medical and procedural or surgical interventions are generally undertaken when more conservative measures have failed or are inappropriate for the patient's particular form of DED. Medical interventions include a variety of topical lubricants, tear film replacements, and immune modulators [9-15]. Surgical and procedural interventions include punctual plugging [16-19], salivary gland transplantation [20-25], limbal grafting [26-29], and partial or complete tarsorrhapy in severe disease. Additional treatment options include using corneal shielding devices [30] and chamber goggles [31] to provide corneal protection or reduce tear film evaporation, respectively.

Currently tear replacement in the form of artificial tears is by far the most widely used therapy for DED, and a wide variety of lubricants have been employed to create the plethora of commercial preparations used in clinical practice. These substitutes should ideally lubricate the ocular surface and decrease evaporation. Preparations contain various cocktails of carboxymethyl cellulose (CMC), hydroxypropyl methylcellulose (HMPC), polyvinyl alcohol (PVA), propylene glycol (PG), glycerin, mineral oil and white petrolatum [32]. Unfortunately, clinical studies have revealed that the majority of commonly used artificial tear preparations are rapidly cleared from the ocular surface and provide little more than 10-20 minutes of lubrication before the tear film returns to the pre-application baseline [33].

An additional problem with artificial tears is the deleterious effects of preservative compounds on the eye, which include conjunctival inflammation, cataract development, corneal toxicity, anterior chamber inflammation, trabecular meshwork damage, and macular edema [34-37].

Preservative-free preparations are available, but are typically more expensive than preserved solutions and come in single-use vials that must be carried by patients to maintain an adequate dosage.

Finally, a commonly cited deficiency of artificial tear preparations is their lack of protein and vitamin content [38], specifically those present in natural tears that are essential for nourishing the ocular surface, promoting regeneration of damaged cornea, and protecting the eye from infection.

BIOLOGICAL PROPERTIES OF SERUM, PLASMA AND NATURAL TEARS

An ocular surface epithelium that demonstrates normal proliferation, differentiation and maturation is an important requirement for maintaining ocular surface health. The normal tear film provides several components that promote these functions, including a stable laminar structure consisting of a thin external lipid phase, a relatively thick (3-4 μm) aqueous phase, and a mucus phase overlying the corneal epithelium, and a complex mixture of growth factors, vitamins, glycoproteins, and antimicrobial molecules within the tear film itself (Table 1).

The protein component of tears is incredibly complex, with the tear proteome containing an estimated 1,543 individual proteins [39]. Among these, several tear-specific proteins, such as lacritin and lipocalin-1, appear to play an important role in the maintenance of tear film stability and basal tearing [40, 41], and are thus considered as desirable components of the native tear film. The role of proinflammatory cytokines and growth factors such as interleukins, TGF-β and EGF in DED remains unclear, with researchers variously reporting beneficial and deleterious effects of these factors during disease pathogenesis and resolution [11, 42-45].

Lactoferrin, the major glycoprotein component in human tears, has potent broad-spectrum antimicrobial activity and is deficient in the tears of individuals with DED [46-49]. Fibronectin, a large glycoprotein also present in tears, plays an important role in wound healing [50] and has been used as a topical agent in the treatment of DED with modest success [51-53]. Lysozyme and IgA are both abundant in tears and provide antimicrobial activity to the eye and other mucosal surfaces [54, 55].

In addition to these components, vitamins A and C are present in tears and promote corneal wound healing and maintenance of the ocular surface [56-59].

Table 1. Comparison of the contents of natural tears and blood serum

	Tears	Serum
pH	7.4	7.4
Osmolarity	298	296
EGF (ng/mL)	0.2–3.0	0.5
TGF-β (ng/mL)	2–10	6–33
Vitamin A (mg/mL)	0.02	46
Vitamin C (mg/mL)	0.117	0.020
Lysozyme (mg/mL)	2.4	0.015
IgA (μg/mL)	411	1500
Fibronectin (μg/mL)	21	205
Lactoferrin (mg/mL)	1.51	Not detected
Transferrin (mg/mL)	Not detected	2

Data from Geerling et al. [100], reproduced with permission.

Autologous Plasma in the Treatment of Dry Eye Disease

Several findings suggest that autologous plasma may be an effective alternative to artificial preparations for the treatment of DED. The use of autologous plasma promotes an improvement in the condition of the corneal surface within 1–2 months of starting treatment (Table 2), as measured by a reduction in corneal fluorescein staining. Such improvements also occur with the use of autologous serum [60, 61], although results may vary depending on the patients' particular presentation and form of disease. This finding clearly demonstrates the efficacy of plasma in the promotion of corneal healing, and is presumably a function of the plasma growth factors mentioned above.

A logical extension of this finding is to determine which components of the plasma milieu are responsible for the observed corneal epithelium healing. Recent clinical trials using topical formulations of specific receptor modulators for growth factors implicated in dry eye disease, including IL-1 and TNFα, have already demonstrated the benefit of such rational approaches to dry eye treatment [62-66].

The frequency of eye drop application is substantially reduced in patients using autologous plasma compared to the same patients using artificial tears (Table 2). Similar reductions in eye drop application occur when autologous serum is used [67].

Table 2. The impact of autologous plasma eyedrops on dry eye signs and symptoms. The 95% confidence intervals are shown in parentheses

Variable	Pre-treatment	Post-treatment	*P*-value
Corneal staining			
Superior	1.8 (0.8 – 2.8)	1.4 (0.5 – 2.3)	0.11
Inferior	3.2 (2.4–4.0)	2.7 (1.9 – 3.5)	0.01*
Temporal	2.6 (1.7 – 3.6)	1.8 (1.2 – 2.4)	0.001*
Nasal	3.2 (2.5–4.0)	2.1 (1.3–2.9)	0.001*
Central	2.5 (1.5–3.5)	1.6 (0.8–2.4)	0.001*
Schirmer distance (mm)	2.1 (1.3 – 3.0)	1.8 (1.1 – 2.6)	0.57
Tear break-up time (s)	3.1 (2.5 – 3.7)	2.6 (2.0 – 3.2)	0.19
Global symptom score	74.2 (66.7 – 81.7)	66.1 (52.5 – 79.6)	0.35
Eyedrop frequency (per day)	12.1 (7.9 – 16.3)	7.3 (4.6 – 9.9)	0.001*
Intraocular pressure (mm Hg)	14.4 (13.0 – 15.8)	15.1 (13.4 – 16.8)	0.34
Visual acuity (logMar)	0.2 (0.1 – 0.4)	0.2 (0.1 – 0.3)	0.17

*These values represent significant improvements in the corneal epithelium and frequency of eyedrop use following the use of autologous plasma, compared to the patient's baseline.

Data from Petznick et al. [75].

This is an important outcome as it suggests an improved quality of life for dry eye patients with less interference of daily activities. Indeed, patient quality of life is significantly affected in moderate DED and has been likened to that of moderate angina [68]. Tear breakup time (TBUT), a measure of the stability of the ocular tear film, has been reported in numerous studies to be lengthened (i.e., improved) by the use of autologous serum eye drops [67, 69-73]. The authors have not observed such improvements when autologous plasma is used, although half of a patient cohort treated with platelet-rich plasma experienced improved TBUT [74]. In our clinical trials patients did not experience a significant reduction of their dry eye symptoms [75]. Another study enrolled patients who experienced dry eye symptoms after undergoing a LASIK procedure also failed to demonstrate any differences in comfort scores with serum treatment [76]. However, the findings in LASIK-induced dry eye may not be comparable to other types of dry eye [77]. Several other investigations noted a significant improvement of dry eye symptoms with the use of autologous serum and some patients reported better ocular comfort within the first 48 hours [67, 69-73].

In these previous reports, dry eye symptoms or pain scores were measured by face scores [69, 71], numerical scores [73, 76] or VAS scores [70]. The reason for the lack of improved dry eye symptoms in our investigations is not clear and may be due to the small sample size, short follow-up period, and expectations of the patients receiving autologous plasma treatment.

Few adverse events in response to autologous serum have been reported. Three out of 203 patients (a rate of 1.5%) had infection as a complication, [78] while other adverse events include eczema around the eyelids [72] and immunoglobulin deposition in the cornea [79].

It should be noted that all of the reported infections occurred in a single study [73]. The three patients had persistent epithelial defects and one had retained sutures from penetrating keratoplasty prior to autologous serum treatment, a high risk factor for infection [80].

These infections appear to have been related to contamination of a dropper bottle [73]. Microbial colonization of the dropper bottle before and after 24 hours of use by patients resulted in almost 10% of bottles testing positive for *Staphylococcus epidermidis* and *S. aureus*, as well as *Streptococcus* and *Micrococcus* species [81]. This highlights the risk of reusing dropper bottles compared to single-use disposable applicators or tubes.

To minimize the risk of contamination we have adopted two approaches: (1) a closed method for preparation and; (2) plasma application using small segments of tubing that are discarded after a single use. Using these two approaches, we found that autologous plasma is convenient to use for treating DED and does not cause discomfort and adverse effects.

Instructions for correct instillation of plasma that avoids direct contact with the eye and prevents subsequent contamination are given to each patient. Randomly selected segments from patients are tested for bacterial and fungal growth by standard culturing techniques. Patients use autologous plasma at least three times daily, amounting to 3–4 segments per day, for six weeks. This follow-up period is ample for the analysis of corneal wound healing, which typically takes place within one to three days and under normal circumstances [82], and was comparable in duration to previous studies [61, 70, 72, 83, 84]. Longer follow-up periods may be desirable for improved assessment of long-term patient adherence, especially given the inconvenience of blood donation and collection. Assays of serum and plasma suggest that these preparations are generally stable at –20°C for three to six months [85-87], necessitating blood collection several times each year.

PREPARATION OF PLASMA FOR USE ON THE OCULAR SURFACE

Contemporary use of plasmapheresis has focused predominantly on its utility in the treatment of autoimmune and immune-mediated diseases, where the removal harmful antibodies from the blood provides a rapid and effective solution for many immunological diseases [88-90]. In the treatment of dry eye disease the goals of therapy are very different to these applications.

As mentioned above, autologous serum contains essential components that are also present in tears and it has been used a tear substitute for patients with DED since the early 1980s [91]. Standard protocols for the preparation of autologous serum have been published [92, 93], although there is still no universally accepted protocol for serum preparation that would reduce the risk of contamination to a minimum. This represents a problem for approval by regulatory bodies and also prevents widespread clinical use.

Autologous serum is generally prepared after collection of blood from the patient by venipuncture. Following removal of clotting factors and dilution with saline, serum preparations are dispensed into containers.

This "open" method of eye drop preparation creates an increased risk of microbial contamination and poses a significant threat of eye infections [73]. An alternative to this method is to prepare autologous plasma in a 'closed' system. In collaboration with transfusion medicine specialists, eye drops may be prepared directly after plasmapheresis without the need for further clotting and dilution steps. Such preparation may expedite regulatory approval and enable incorporation of this modality into clinical practice.

In our approach, plasma collection from DED patients is undertaken using an automated continuous filtration plasma collection system (MCS+, Haemonetics, Massachusetts, US) in collaboration with clinical hematologists. Under ideal conditions, approximately 500–600 mL of plasma can be collected in 30–40 minutes using this approach. Prior to collection, patient blood parameters including a full blood count with differential, prothrombin and activated partial thromboplastin times, and serum electrolytes are assessed, although abnormalities do not necessarily preclude plasma collection. Plasma is collected from each subject in a sealed container over a 30 minute period and drained into intravenous-grade 4 mm tubing, which is then crimped into short segments using an automated multi-head radio-frequency-based crimper (Genesis SE530, Genesis Packaging Technologies, Nyon, Switzerland).

Each segment contains 150–300 μL of plasma. This method of sealing the tubes is advantageous as there is no leakage even if single sealed segments are separated from the rest of the crimped tubing. In our current treatment protocol, we employ the services of a clinical hematology center, and are able to benefit from the use of trained hematology personnel for pre-screening, plasmapheresis procedures, storage if necessary, and dispensing of plasma to dry eye patients.

High dilutions of autologous serum were initially thought to be harmful to the sensitive balance of the ocular surface system [69]. Several components in serum, including TGF-β and vitamin A, are substantially more concentrated than they are in tears (Table 1). However, when applied to the ocular surface, higher concentrations of serum support corneal cell migration better than lower concentrations [92]. This has been attributed to the higher concentrations of the migration-promoting component fibronectin [92]. A major problem faced by proponents of serum eye drops, however, is the time-consuming and meticulous protocols required to prepare useful volumes of therapeutic serum. One approach is to begin therapy with diluted serum and increase serum concentrations if a patient's clinical response is inadequate [61, 92]. It remains to be seen if this approach is effective with autologous plasma, although the addition of extra procedural steps inevitably increases the production cost and contamination risk of this already expensive process.

Following preparation of the plasma-filled tubes, patients can be given the preparation in a zip-lock bag or plastic container, which is then stored in their household freezer at –20°C. Alternatively, the freshly collected plasma can be stored in the collection center at –80°C and dispensed at a later date. This may be desirable if the collection center needs to perform serological screens on the plasma prior to dispensing to the patient. When the plasma is needed, patients twist off the desired number of segments and defrost them in a refrigerator at 4°C. Each segment ideally contains sufficient plasma for both eyes and is applied without contacting the eye, and then discarded after use.

REGULATIONS, SAFETY AND ETHICAL CONSIDERATIONS

Plasmapheresis procedures have dramatically improved in recent years following the introduction of modern chromatography methods and effective removal of infectious agents, increasing both the quality and safety of plasma products [94].

The reliability of current plasmapheresis methods prompted the authors to explore this is an alternative to artificial tears and autologous serum preparations for the treatment of dry eye disease. As with all biological therapeutics, however, the use of plasma necessitates the consideration of ethical and safety issues before it may be adopted in a large-scale fashion outside of small clinical trials.

Despite the substantial benefits to dry eye patients, autologous serum and plasma are not widely used. This is likely due to a combination of poorly standardized preparation protocols, cumbersome preparation methods, clinician knowledge, and patient preferences. To date there has been no formal approval granted by regulatory bodies, including the American Food and Drug Administration, for the use of autologous plasma to treat ocular surface disorders. Standardized protocols for the preparation of autologous serum eye drops have been proposed and even implemented in the United Kingdom, albeit with an unsubsidized cost of more than US$2,000 per donation episode [92, 95]. Among developed nations, relatively few medical centers are licensed to produce autologous serum for use as eye drops [96].

The advantage offered by plasmapheresis is that relatively few alterations need to be made to existing well-established plasmapheresis protocols currently in use in most tertiary hospitals. Also, the risk of contamination with airborne pathogens during the preparation of serum eye drops from whole blood in the open systems described previously [92] are circumvented by using a closed circuit plasmapheresis system as described above.

These advantages will enable the rapid establishment of a set of standards for autologous plasma eye drop preparation if clinical interest remains strong.

Despite these advantages, not all patients are suitable candidates for plasmapheresis. They may have medical conditions such as blood-borne viral infections or allergies to the anticoagulants used in plasmapheresis which preclude the use autologous plasma for treatment of their DED.

Allogeneic plasma donated by relatives is an option in such cases, but this raises additional ethical dilemmas. Previous reports on the use of autologous serum or plasma for DED have incorporated screening for HIV, HBV, HCV, and syphilis into production protocols [75, 84, 93].

Disease screening is of paramount importance when donor blood products are used for DED. At least one case of HIV transmission via a single infected drop of serum being splashed into the eye has been reported in the literature [97].

Another major infection risk for eye drops prepared from allogeneic blood occurs when blood is taken from a HIV-positive individual during the window period of HIV infection when the virus remains undetectable by conventional testing methods [98], although no infections via ocular inoculation of such a sample have yet been reported in the literature.

Most hospital transfusion services knowingly store and transfuse autologous blood and autologous blood products that are untested or test positive for infectious disease, with almost half of US transfusion services storing HIV-positive autologous blood with special authorization [99].

Such practices carry a risk of mis-transfusion of infected blood into uninfected patients. It is important to point out, however, that this is not an issue for plasmapheresis eye drops because they are prepared and dispensed to the patient in a single session on the same day with no intermediate storage required.

Moreover, the preparation of autologous plasma in a closed-circuit system virtually precludes the introduction of exogenous pathogens into the final product, although there is potential for blood-borne pathogens that did not previously have access to the ocular surface to be introduced via eye drops and cause infection. This route of transmission has not yet been documented, though a theoretical risk remains.

CONCLUSION

The social and economic burden of dry eye disease is considerable and improved treatment options that address both the symptoms and underlying disease process have not yet become widely available. Autologous plasma provides an alternative treatment option to conventional artificial tear solutions and shows efficacy in treating the damage that occurs to the corneal epithelium during prolonged dry eye disease.

Although the use of serum and plasma has previously been limited by regulatory restrictions and cumbersome preparation methods that carry risks of product contamination, it is possible to avoid these problems by utilizing existing high-throughput plasmapheresis equipment and clinical hematology staff for the preparation of autologous plasma.

Patients can store eyedrops prepared in this way for extended periods and require less frequent application than conventional artificial tear treatments.

ACKNOWLEDGMENTS

We thank Dr. William Hwang, Head and Senior Consultant, Department of Haematology, Singapore General Hospital, for his input.

REFERENCES

[1] The definition and classification of dry eye disease: report of the Definition and Classification Subcommittee of the International Dry Eye WorkShop (2007). *Ocul. Surf.* 2007, 5:75–92.

[2] Rege, A., Kulkarni, V., Puthran, N., Khandgave, T.: A Clinical Study of Subtype-based Prevalence of Dry Eye. *J. Clin. Diagn. Res. JCDR* 2013, 7:2207–2210.

[3] Schiffman, R. M., Christianson, M. D., Jacobsen, G., Hirsch, J. D., Reis, B. L.: Reliability and validity of the Ocular Surface Disease Index. *Arch. Ophthalmol.* 2000, 118:615–621.

[4] Lee, A. J., Lee, J., Saw, S.-M., Gazzard, G., Koh, D., Widjaja, D., Tan, D. T. H.: Prevalence and risk factors associated with dry eye symptoms: a population based study in Indonesia. *Br. J. Ophthalmol.* 2002, 86: 1347–1351.

[5] Mizuno, Y., Yamada, M., Shigeyasu, C.: Annual direct cost of dry eye in Japan. *Clin. Ophthalmol. Auckl. NZ* 2012, 6:755–760.

[6] Yamada, M., Mizuno, Y., Shigeyasu, C.: Impact of dry eye on work productivity. *Clin. Outcomes Res. CEOR* 2012, 4:307–312.

[7] Waduthantri, S., Yong, S. S., Tan, C. H., Shen, L., Lee, M. X., Nagarajan, S., Hla, M. H., Tong, L.: Cost of Dry Eye Treatment in an Asian Clinic Setting [Internet]. *PLoS ONE* 2012, 7.

[8] Yu, J., Asche, C. V., Fairchild, C. J.: The economic burden of dry eye disease in the United States: a decision tree analysis. *Cornea* 2011, 30: 379–387.

[9] Chung, Y. W., Oh, T. H., Chung, S. K.: The effect of topical cyclosporine 0.05% on dry eye after cataract surgery. *Korean J. Ophthalmol. KJO* 2013, 27:167–171.

[10] Hoehn, M. E., Kelly, S. R., Wilson, M. W., Walton, R. C.: Cyclosporine 0.05% ophthalmic emulsion for the treatment of radiation-associated dry eye in children. *Pediatr. Blood Cancer* 2013, 60:E35–37.

[11] Lee, H. S., Jang, J. Y., Lee, S. H., Im, S. K., Yoon, K. C.: Clinical effectiveness of topical cyclosporine a 0.05% after laser epithelial keratomileusis. *Cornea* 2013, 32:e150–155.

[12] Pérez-Rico, C., Germain, F., Castro-Rebollo, M., Moreno-Salgueiro, A., Teus, M. Á.: Effect of topical 0.05% cyclosporine A on corneal endothelium in patients with dry eye disease. *Int. J. Ophthalmol.* 2013, 6:471–474.

[13] Prabhasawat, P., Tesavibul, N., Karnchanachetanee, C., Kasemson, S.: Efficacy of cyclosporine 0.05% eye drops in Stevens Johnson syndrome with chronic dry eye. *J. Ocul. Pharmacol. Ther. Off. J. Assoc. Ocul. Pharmacol. Ther.* 2013, 29:372–377.

[14] Prabhasawat, P., Tesavibul, N., Mahawong, W.: A randomized double-masked study of 0.05% cyclosporine ophthalmic emulsion in the treatment of meibomian gland dysfunction. *Cornea* 2012, 31:1386–1393.

[15] Sanz-Marco, E., Udaondo, P., García-Delpech, S., Vazquez, A., Diaz-Llopis, M.: Treatment of refractory dry eye associated with graft versus host disease with 0.03% tacrolimus eyedrops. *J. Ocul. Pharmacol. Ther. Off. J. Assoc. Ocul. Pharmacol. Ther.* 2013, 29:776–783.

[16] Qiu, W., Liu, Z., Ao, M., Li, X., Wang, W.: Punctal plugs versus artificial tears for treating primary Sjögren's syndrome with kerato-conjunctivitis SICCA: a comparative observation of their effects on visual function. *Rheumatol. Int.* 2013, 33:2543–2548.

[17] Rabensteiner, D. F., Boldin, I., Klein, A., Horwath-Winter, J.: Collared silicone punctal plugs compared to intracanalicular plugs for the treatment of dry eye. *Curr. Eye Res.* 2013, 38:521–525.

[18] Kaido, M., Ishida, R., Dogru, M., Tsubota, K.: Comparison of retention rates and complications of 2 different types of silicon lacrimal punctal plugs in the treatment of dry eye disease. *Am. J. Ophthalmol.* 2013, 155: 648–653, 653.e1.

[19] Chi, S. L., Acquah, K. F., Richard, M. J., Lee, P. P., Sloan, F. A.: Longitudinal evidence on punctal plug use in an elderly population. *Ophthal. Plast. Reconstr. Surg.* 2012, 28:289–293.

[20] Geerling, G., Collin, J. R. O., Dart, J. K. G.: Ophthalmic experience with submandibular gland transplantation for severe dry eyes. *The Laryngoscope* 2009, 119:1445–1446.

[21] Sant' Anna, A. E. B. P. P., Hazarbassanov, R. M., de Freitas, D., Gomes, J. Á. P.: Minor salivary glands and labial mucous membrane graft in the

treatment of severe symblepharon and dry eye in patients with Stevens-Johnson syndrome. *Br. J. Ophthalmol.* 2012, 96:234–239.

[22] Qin, J., Zhang, L., Cai, Z., Mao, C., Liu, X., Lv, L., Zou, L., Peng, X., Su, J., Wu, J., et al.: Microvascular autologous transplantation of partial submandibular gland for severe keratoconjunctivitis sicca. *Br. J. Ophthalmol.* 2013, 97:1123–1128.

[23] Su, J., Liu, X., Zhang, L., Yu, G.: Schirmer test in transplanted submandibular gland: influencing factors and a modified measurement method. *Cornea* 2013, 32:419–422.

[24] Geerling, G., Sieg, P.: Transplantation of the major salivary glands. *Dev. Ophthalmol.* 2008, 41:255–268.

[25] Chen, Z., Jie, Y., Yu, G.: Treatment of severe keratoconjunctivitis sicca by parotid duct transposition after tympanic neurectomy in rabbits. *Invest. Ophthalmol. Vis. Sci.* 2011, 52:6964–6970.

[26] Santos, M. S., Gomes, J. A. P., Hofling-Lima, A. L., Rizzo, L. V., Romano, A. C., Belfort, R. Jr: Survival analysis of conjunctival limbal grafts and amniotic membrane transplantation in eyes with total limbal stem cell deficiency. *Am. J. Ophthalmol.* 2005, 140:223–230.

[27] Holland, E. J., Schwartz, G. S.: The evolution of epithelial transplantation for severe ocular surface disease and a proposed classification system. *Cornea* 1996, 15:549–556.

[28] Holland, E. J., Schwartz, G. S.: Changing concepts in the management of severe ocular surface disease over twenty-five years. *Cornea* 2000, 19:688–698.

[29] Dua, H. S., Miri, A., Said, D. G.: Contemporary limbal stem cell transplantation - a review. *Clin. Experiment. Ophthalmol.* 2010, 38:104–117.

[30] Hayworth, N. A., Asbell, P. A.: Therapeutic contact lenses. *CLAO J. Off. Publ. Contact Lens Assoc. Ophthalmol. Inc* 1990, 16:137–142.

[31] Korb, D. R., Blackie, C. A.: Using goggles to increase periocular humidity and reduce dry eye symptoms. *Eye Contact Lens* 2013, 39: 273–276.

[32] Dogru, M., Nakamura, M., Shimazaki, J., Tsubota, K.: Changing trends in the treatment of dry-eye disease. *Expert Opin. Investig. Drugs* 2013, doi:10.1517/13543784.2013.838557.

[33] Wang, J., Simmons, P., Aquavella, J., Vehige, J., Palakuru, J., Chung, S., Feng, C.: Dynamic distribution of artificial tears on the ocular surface. *Arch. Ophthalmol.* 2008, 126:619–625.

[34] Paimela, T., Ryhänen, T., Kauppinen, A., Marttila, L., Salminen, A., Kaarniranta, K.: The preservative polyquaternium-1 increases cytoxicity

and NF-kappaB linked inflammation in human corneal epithelial cells. *Mol. Vis.* 2012, 18:1189–1196.

[35] Whitson, J. T., Petroll, W. M.: Corneal epithelial cell viability following exposure to ophthalmic solutions containing preservatives and/or antihypertensive agents. *Adv. Ther.* 2012, 29:874–888.

[36] Okahara, A., Kawazu, K.: Local toxicity of benzalkonium chloride in ophthalmic solutions following repeated applications. *J. Toxicol. Sci.* 2013, 38:531–537.

[37] Rosin, L. M., Bell, N. P.: Preservative toxicity in glaucoma medication: clinical evaluation of benzalkonium chloride-free 0.5% timolol eye drops. *Clin. Ophthalmol. Auckl. NZ* 2013, 7:2131–2135.

[38] Holland, E. J., Mannis, M. J., Lee, W. Barry: *Ocular Surface Disease: Cornea, Conjunctiva and Tear Film.* Elsevier; 2013.

[39] Zhou, L., Zhao, S. Z., Koh, S. K., Chen, L., Vaz, C., Tanavde, V., Li, X. R., Beuerman, R. W.: In-depth analysis of the human tear proteome. *J. Proteomics* 2012, 75:3877–3885.

[40] Karnati, R., Laurie, D. E., Laurie, G. W.: Lacritin and the tear proteome as natural replacement therapy for dry eye. *Exp. Eye Res.* 2013, 117:39–52.

[41] Fujii, A., Morimoto-Tochigi, A., Walkup, R. D., Shearer, T. R., Azuma, M.: Lacritin-induced secretion of tear proteins from cultured monkey lacrimal acinar cells. *Invest. Ophthalmol. Vis. Sci.* 2013, 54:2533–2540.

[42] Benito, M. J., Calder, V., Corrales, R. M., García-Vázquez, C., Narayanan, S., Herreras, J. M., Stern, M. E., Calonge, M., Enríquez-de-Salamanca, A.: Effect of TGF-β on ocular surface epithelial cells. *Exp. Eye Res.* 2013, 107:88–100.

[43] De Paiva, C. S., Volpe, E. A., Gandhi, N. B., Zhang, X., Zheng, X., Pitcher, J. D. 3rd, Farley, W. J., Stern, M. E., Niederkorn, J. Y., Li, D.-Q., et al.: Disruption of TGF-β signaling improves ocular surface epithelial disease in experimental autoimmune keratoconjunctivitis sicca. *PloS One* 2011, 6:e29017.

[44] Rao, K., Farley, W. J., Pflugfelder, S. C.: Association between high tear epidermal growth factor levels and corneal subepithelial fibrosis in dry eye conditions. *Invest. Ophthalmol. Vis. Sci.* 2010, 51:844–849.

[45] Enríquez-de-Salamanca, A., Castellanos, E., Stern, M. E., Fernández, I., Carreño, E., García-Vázquez, C., Herreras, J. M., Calonge, M.: Tear cytokine and chemokine analysis and clinical correlations in evaporative-type dry eye disease. *Mol. Vis.* 2010, 16:862–873.

[46] Ohashi, Y., Ishida, R., Kojima, T., Goto, E., Matsumoto, Y., Watanabe, K., Ishida, N., Nakata, K., Takeuchi, T., Tsubota, K.: Abnormal protein profiles in tears with dry eye syndrome. *Am. J. Ophthalmol.* 2003, 136: 291–299.

[47] Versura, P., Nanni, P., Bavelloni, A., Blalock, W. L., Piazzi, M., Roda, A., Campos, E. C.: Tear proteomics in evaporative dry eye disease. *Eye Lond. Engl.* 2010, 24:1396–1402.

[48] Flanagan, J. L., Willcox, M. D. P.: Role of lactoferrin in the tear film. *Biochimie* 2009, 91:35–43.

[49] Versura, P., Bavelloni, A., Grillini, M., Fresina, M., Campos, E. C.: Diagnostic performance of a tear protein panel in early dry eye. *Mol. Vis.* 2013, 19:1247–1257.

[50] Pankov, R., Yamada, K. M.: Fibronectin at a glance. *J. Cell Sci.* 2002, 115:3861–3863.

[51] Nishida, T.: Translational research in corneal epithelial wound healing. *Eye Contact Lens* 2010, 36:300–304.

[52] Kono, I., Matsumoto, Y., Kono, K., Ishibashi, Y., Narushima, K., Kabashima, T., Yamane, K., Sakurai, T., Kashiwagi, H.: Beneficial effect of topical fibronectin in patients with keratoconjunctivitis sicca of Sjögren's syndrome. *J. Rheumatol.* 1985, 12:487–489.

[53] Nelson, J. D., Gordon, J. F.: Topical fibronectin in the treatment of kera toconjunctivitis sicca. Chiron Keratoconjunctivitis Sicca Study Group. *Am. J. Ophthalmol.* 1992, 114:441–447.

[54] Franklin, R. M.: The ocular secretory immune system: a review. *Curr. Eye Res.* 1989, 8:599–606.

[55] McClellan, K. A.: Mucosal defense of the outer eye. *Surv. Ophthalmol.* 1997, 42:233–246.

[56] Kim, E. C., Choi, J.-S., Joo, C.-K.: A comparison of vitamin a and cyclosporine a 0.05% eye drops for treatment of dry eye syndrome. *Am. J. Ophthalmol.* 2009, 147:206–213.e3.

[57] Selek, H., Unlü, N., Orhan, M., Irkeç, M.: Evaluation of retinoic acid ophthalmic emulsion in dry eye. *Eur. J. Ophthalmol.* 2000, 10:121–127.

[58] Peponis, V., Bonovas, S., Kapranou, A., Peponi, E., Filioussi, K., Magkou, C., Sitaras, N. M.: Conjunctival and tear film changes after vitamin C and E administration in non-insulin dependent diabetes mellitus. *Med. Sci. Monit. Int. Med. J. Exp. Clin. Res.* 2004, 10:CR213–217.

[59] Choy, C. K. M., Benzie, I. F. F., Cho, P.: Is ascorbate in human tears from corneal leakage or from lacrimal secretion? *Clin. Exp. Optom. J. Aust. Optom. Assoc.* 2004, 87:24–27.

[60] Pan, Q., Angelina, A., Zambrano, A., Marrone, M., Stark, W. J., Heflin, T., Tang, L., Akpek, E. K.: Autologous serum eye drops for dry eye. *Cochrane Database Syst. Rev.* 2013, 8:CD009327.

[61] Urzua, C. A., Vasquez, D. H., Huidobro, A., Hernandez, H., Alfaro, J.: Randomized double-blind clinical trial of autologous serum versus artificial tears in dry eye syndrome. *Curr. Eye Res.* 2012, 37:684–688.

[62] Amparo, F., Dastjerdi, M. H., Okanobo, A., Ferrari, G., Smaga, L., Hamrah, P., Jurkunas, U., Schaumberg, D. A., Dana, R.: Topical interleukin 1 receptor antagonist for treatment of dry eye disease: a randomized clinical trial. *JAMA Ophthalmol.* 2013, 131:715–723.

[63] Meerovitch, K., Torkildsen, G., Lonsdale, J., Goldfarb, H., Lama, T., Cumberlidge, G., Ousler, G. W. 3rd: Safety and efficacy of MIM-D3 ophthalmic solutions in a randomized, placebo-controlled Phase 2 clinical trial in patients with dry eye. *Clin. Ophthalmol. Auckl. NZ* 2013, 7: 1275–1285.

[64] Hou, J., Townson, S. A., Kovalchin, J. T., Masci, A., Kiner, O., Shu, Y., King, B. M., Schirmer, E., Golden, K., Thomas, C., et al.: Design of a superior cytokine antagonist for topical ophthalmic use. *Proc. Natl. Acad. Sci. US.* 2013, 110:3913–3918.

[65] Okanobo, A., Chauhan, S. K., Dastjerdi, M. H., Kodati, S., Dana, R.: Efficacy of topical blockade of interleukin-1 in experimental dry eye disease. *Am. J. Ophthalmol.* 2012, 154:63–71.

[66] Li, Z., Choi, W., Oh, H.-J., Yoon, K. C.: Effectiveness of topical infliximab in a mouse model of experimental dry eye. *Cornea* 2012, 31 Suppl. 1:S25–31.

[67] Tananuvat, N., Daniell, M., Sullivan, L. J., Yi, Q., McKelvie, P., McCarty, D. J., Taylor, H. R.: Controlled study of the use of autologous serum in dry eye patients. *Cornea* 2001, 20:802–806.

[68] Buchholz, P., Steeds, C. S., Stern, L. S., Wiederkehr, D. P., Doyle, J. J., Katz, L. M., Figueiredo, F. C.: Utility assessment to measure the impact of dry eye disease. *Ocul. Surf.* 2006, 4:155–161.

[69] Tsubota, K., Goto, E., Fujita, H., Ono, M., Inoue, H., Saito, I., Shimmura, S.: Treatment of dry eye by autologous serum application in Sjögren's syndrome. *Br. J. Ophthalmol.* 1999, 83:390–395.

[70] Kojima, T., Ishida, R., Dogru, M., Goto, E., Matsumoto, Y., Kaido, M., Tsubota, K.: The effect of autologous serum eyedrops in the treatment of

severe dry eye disease: a prospective randomized case-control study. *Am. J. Ophthalmol.* 2005, 139:242–246.
[71] Noble, B. A., Loh, R. S. K., MacLennan, S., Pesudovs, K., Reynolds, A., Bridges, L. R., Burr, J., Stewart, O., Quereshi, S.: Comparison of autologous serum eye drops with conventional therapy in a randomised controlled crossover trial for ocular surface disease. *Br. J. Ophthalmol.* 2004, 88:647–652.
[72] Ogawa, Y., Okamoto, S., Mori, T., Yamada, M., Mashima, Y., Watanabe, R., Kuwana, M., Tsubota, K., Ikeda, Y., Oguchi, Y.: Autologous serum eye drops for the treatment of severe dry eye in patients with chronic graft-versus-host disease. *Bone Marrow Transplant.* 2003, 31: 579–583.
[73] Poon, A. C., Geerling, G., Dart, J. K., Fraenkel, G. E., Daniels, J. T.: Autologous serum eyedrops for dry eyes and epithelial defects: clinical and in vitro toxicity studies. *Br. J. Ophthalmol.* 2001, 85:1188–1197.
[74] Alio, J. L., Colecha, J. R., Pastor, S., Rodriguez, A., Artola, A.: Symptomatic dry eye treatment with autologous platelet-rich plasma. *Ophthalmic Res.* 2007, 39:124–129.
[75] Petznick, A., Tong, L., Chung, R., Wang, J. C., Koh, M., Salleh, R., Waduthantri, S.: Autologous plasma eyedrops prepared in a closed system: a treatment for dry eye. *Eye Lond. Engl.* 2013, 27:1102.
[76] Noda-Tsuruya, T., Asano-Kato, N., Toda, I., Tsubota, K.: Autologous serum eye drops for dry eye after LASIK. *J. Refract. Surg. Thorofare NJ* 1995 2006, 22:61–66.
[77] Patel, S. V., McLaren, J. W., Kittleson, K. M., Bourne, W. M.: Subbasal nerve density and corneal sensitivity after laser in situ keratomileusis: femtosecond laser vs mechanical microkeratome. *Arch. Ophthalmol.* 2010, 128:1413–1419.
[78] Yamada, C., King, K. E., Ness, P. M.: Autologous serum eyedrops: literature review and implications for transfusion medicine specialists. *Transfusion (Paris)* 2008, 48:1245–1255.
[79] McDonnell, P. J., Schanzlin, D. J., Rao, N. A.: Immunoglobulin deposition in the cornea after application of autologous serum. *Arch. Ophthalmol.* 1988, 106:1423–1425.
[80] Varley, G. A., Meisler, D. M.: Complications of penetrating keratoplasty: graft infections. *Refract. Corneal Surg.* 1991, 7:62–66.
[81] Lagnado, R., King, A. J., Donald, F., Dua, H. S.: A protocol for low contamination risk of autologous serum drops in the management of ocular surface disorders. *Br. J. Ophthalmol.* 2004, 88:464–465.

[82] Dua, H. S., Forrester, J. V.: Clinical patterns of corneal epithelial wound healing. *Am. J. Ophthalmol.* 1987, 104:481–489.

[83] Matsumoto, Y., Dogru, M., Goto, E., Ohashi, Y., Kojima, T., Ishida, R., Tsubota, K.: Autologous serum application in the treatment of neurotrophic keratopathy. *Ophthalmology* 2004, 111:1115–1120.

[84] Partal, A., Scott, E.: Low-cost protocol for the production of autologous serum eye drops by blood collection and processing centres for the treatment of ocular surface diseases. *Transfus. Med. Oxf. Engl.* 2011, 21: 271–277.

[85] Fischer, K. R., Opitz, A., Böeck, M., Geerling, G.: Stability of serum eye drops after storage of 6 months. *Cornea* 2012, 31:1313–1318.

[86] Zander, J., Bruegel, M., Kleinhempel, A., Becker, S., Petros, S., Kortz, L., Dorow, J., Kratzsch, J., Baber, R., Ceglarek, U., et al.: Effect of biobanking conditions on short-term stability of biomarkers in human serum and plasma. *Clin. Chem. Lab. Med. CCLM FESCC* 2013, doi:10.1515/cclm-2013-0705.

[87] Anitua, E., Muruzabal, F., Pino, A., Merayo-Lloves, J., Orive, G.: Biological Stability of Plasma Rich in Growth Factors Eye Drops After Storage of 3 Months. *Cornea* 2013, doi:10.1097/ICO.0b013e31829f7088.

[88] Nguyen, T. C., Kiss, J. E., Goldman, J. R., Carcillo, J. A.: The role of plasmapheresis in critical illness. *Crit. Care Clin.* 2012, 28:453–468, vii.

[89] McLeod, B. C.: Plasma and plasma derivatives in therapeutic plasmapheresis. *Transfusion (Paris)* 2012, 52 Suppl. 1:38S–44S.

[90] Pusey, C. D., Levy, J. B.: Plasmapheresis in immunologic renal disease. *Blood Purif.* 2012, 33:190–198.

[91] Fox, R. I., Chan, R., Michelson, J. B., Belmont, J. B., Michelson, P. E.: Beneficial effect of artificial tears made with autologous serum in patients with keratoconjunctivitis sicca. *Arthritis Rheum.* 1984, 27:459–461.

[92] Liu, L., Hartwig, D., Harloff, S., Herminghaus, P., Wedel, T., Geerling, G.: An optimised protocol for the production of autologous serum eyedrops. *Graefes Arch. Clin. Exp. Ophthalmol. Albrecht Von Graefes Arch. Für Klin. Exp. Ophthalmol.* 2005, 243:706–714.

[93] Geerling, G., Maclennan, S., Hartwig, D.: Autologous serum eye drops for ocular surface disorders. *Br. J. Ophthalmol.* 2004, 88:1467–1474.

[94] Burnouf, T.: [Plasma fractionation in the world: current status]. *Transfus. Clin. Biol. J. Société Fr. Transfus. Sang.* 2007, 14:41–50.

[95] Maclennan, S., Hartwig, D., Geerling, G.: [Experiences with a centralised national service for autologous serum eyedrops in England]. *Ophthalmol. Z. Dtsch. Ophthalmol. Ges.* 2008, 105:639–643.

[96] Kasper, K., Godenschweger, L., Hartwig, D., Unterlauft, J. D., Seitz, B., Geerling, G.: [On the use of autologous serum eyedrops in Germany : results of a survey among members of the Cornea Section of the German Ophthalmological Society (DOG)]. *Ophthalmol. Z. Dtsch. Ophthalmol. Ges.* 2008, 105:644–649.

[97] Eberle, J., Habermann, J., Gürtler, L. G.: HIV-1 infection transmitted by serum droplets into the eye: a case report. *AIDS Lond. Engl.* 2000, 14: 206–207.

[98] Müller, B., Nübling, C. M., Kress, J., Roth, W. K., De Zolt, S., Pichl, L.: How safe is safe: new human immunodeficiency virus Type 1 variants missed by nucleic acid testing. *Transfusion (Paris)* 2013, 53:2422–2430.

[99] Shulman, I. A., Osby, M.: Storage and transfusion of infected autologous blood or components: a survey of North American laboratories. *Arch. Pathol. Lab. Med.* 2005, 129:981–983.

[100] Geerling, G., Honnicke, K., Schröder, C., Framme, C., Sieg, P., Lauer, I., Pagel, H., Kirschstein, M., Seyfarth, M., Marx, A. M., et al.: Quality of salivary tears following autologous submandibular gland transplanttation for severe dry eye. *Graefes Arch. Clin. Exp. Ophthalmol. Albrecht Von Graefes Arch. Für Klin. Exp. Ophthalmol.* 2000, 238:45–52.

In: Plasmapheresis and Intravenous ... ISBN: 978-1-63117-916-7
Editor: Rossana Allegro

Chapter 8

SIDE EFFECTS OF INTRAVENOUS IMMUNOGLOBULINS (IVIG)

Krasimir Nikolov*, Milena Nikolova–Vlahova and Marta Baleva

University Hospital Alexandrovska, Medical University, Sofia, Bulgaria

ABSTRACT

During the past decades intravenous immunoglobulins (IVIG) have gained more and more popularity for the treatment of a wide range of diseases and conditions. This treatment is extensively used in immune deficits, autoimmune thrombocytopenia, Kawasaki's disease, for the prevention of infectious complications due to hypogammaglobulinaemia secondary to myeloma, chronic lymphatic leukaemia and post-bone marrow and stem cell transplantation, in Guillain-Barre syndrome, etc. Fewer studies have investigated the use of IVIG in patients with systemic lupus erythematosus (SLE), rheumatoid arthritis, dermatomyositis, multiple sclerosis, myasthenia gravis, in women with reproductive failure, etc.

The wide use of IVIG for the treatment of different diseases and conditions has lead to the emergence of multiple adverse reactions. The large majority of these side effects develop either immediately after the infusion, or within the next 24 hours: reactions at the site of

* Corresponding author: Dr. Krasimir Nikolov, MD, PhD, University Hospital Alexandrovska, 1 G. Sofiiski Str., 1431 Sofia, Bulgaria. Email: krasi@doctor.com.

administration (erythema and rash, itching), tachycardia and low blood pressure, nausea and vomiting, headache, joint and muscle pain, lower back pain, fever, hemolytic reactions, neutropenia, pulmonary edema, deep vein thromboses, etc. There are multiple causes for the development of these side effects, i.e., improper administration of IVIG for inappropriate patients/diseases, rapid intravenous infusion, large quantities of infused IVIG, lack of monitoring during the infusion, the presence of stabilizers and preservatives, sucrose, aggregates, small quantities of IgA or other biological substances and adulterants. An important factor for the prevention of these reactions is the strict attendance to the mode of administration of IVIG, the precise evaluation of the indications for IVIG treatment in every patient and the careful monitoring of the treatment in hospital conditions.

Keywords: Intravenous immunoglobulins (IVIG); treatment; side effects

INTRODUCTION

The treatment with intravenous immunoglobulins (IVIG) has been used for the treatment of different diseases and conditions for more than 50 years. The first reports on the use of IVIG were in patients with immune deficits and chronic lymphoid leukemia. At first, IVIG were administered via intramuscular injections (IM) and more recently the IV and subcutaneous (SC) route is used.

The *in vitro* and *in vivo* studies have revealed the following mechanisms of action of IVIG in autoimmune diseases [1]: Fc receptor blockade, idiotype-anti-idiotype interactions, neutralization of bacteria, toxins and superantigens, competitive inhibition of complement activation, down-regulation of B- and T-cell function, enhancement of pathogenic autoantibodies clearance, modulation of soluble products, apoptosis blockade via Fas receptor and administration of soluble products which could interfere with the immune response.

The US Food and Drug Administration (FDA) and the EU European Medicines Agency (EMA) have approved the following 6 indications for the use of IVIG [2]: 1. For the treatment of primary immune deficiency disorders (PIDD); 2. For the prevention and control of bleeding in idiopathic thrombocytopenic purpura (ITP); 3. For the prevention of coronary aneurisms in Kawasaki's disease; 4. For the treatment of chronic inflammatory demyelinating polyneuropathy; 5. In chronic B-cell lymphocytic leukemia – for the prevention of infectious complications; 6. For the prevention of infectious complications in patient with hypogammaglobulinemia and/or bacterial infections.

Many other indications have been stated in controlled and uncontrolled studies, case reports, clinical guidelines, consensus statements [3-14]. The US FDA states that IVIG treatment also has well documented positive effects in [3]: HIV infection in children for prevention of bacterial infections and hospitalizations and in order to prolong the periods free of serious bacterial infections; in bone marrow transplant recipients > 20 years of age – in order to decrease the risk of septicemia and other infections, interstitial pneumonia and acute graft versus host disease (GVHD) within the first 100 days after the transplantation; in kidney transplant recipients with a high antibody titer or an ABO-incompatible donor; and in multifocal motorneuropathy [4]. Many countries have developed national guidelines (UK [9] and France [10]) and consensus statements (Canada [11, 12] and Australia [13]) for the use of IVIG. Beyond the scope of these well known indications, IVIG are used successfully for the treatment of a wide range of disease: autoimmune (Graves ophthalmopathy, dermatomyositis, polymiositis, severe rheumatoid arthritis, autoimmune diabetes mellitus, autoimmune neutropenia, autoimmune hemolytic anemia, systemic lupus, antiphospholipid syndrome in pregnancy, etc.); neuroimmunologic disorders (Guillain-Barre syndrome, myasthenia gravis, Lambert-Eaton syndrome, multiple sclerosis); in sepsis, septic shock and toxic shock syndrome [3, 4]. More than 150 indications for off-label use of IVIG have been published – many of them as case reports and uncontrolled studies [5]. IVIG have been used as alternative approach in patients with autoimmune diseases who have contraindications for or intolerance to or have no effect on conventional immunosuppressive treatment.

SIDE EFFECTS OF THE IVG TREATMENT

The wide use of IVIG in a large number of immune mediated disorders and immune deficits has led to the emergence of multiple adverse reactions. IVIG are generally well tolerated with the majority of adverse reactions to the medication being mild or moderate and transient with rapid resolution upon cessation of infusion. These reactions include headache, abdominal or back pain, rhinitis, fever, nausea/vomiting, chills, myalgias, wheezing. More serious adverse reactions include: thromboembolic events, hemolysis, renal failure, aseptic meningitis, anaphylactic reactions, hepatitis. According to their severity, V. M. Brennan et al. classify the side effects of IVIG into the following three groups [6]:

1. Mild reactions – headache, flushing, muscle aches, shivering, feeling sick, itching, urticaria, anxiety, lightheadedness, dizziness or irritability. Usually these reactions subside after the cessation of the infusion.
2. Moderate reactions – more severe clinical course of the mild reactions described above, or the emergence of chest pain or wheezing that require cessation of the infusion.
3. Severe reactions – persistent and worsening moderate reactions of the appearance of tightness of the throat, severe headache and shaking, severe breathlessness or wheezing, severe dizziness or fainting, sensation of pressure in the chest or collapse, thromboembolic events, hemolysis, renal failure, aseptic meningitis, anaphylactic reactions, hepatitis. These reactions require immediate cessation of the infusion and the administration of corticosteroids and/or epinephrine.

IVIG are frequently administered in patients with primary immune deficiencies and therefore the vast majority of side effects reported are in these conditions. According to a study performed by the Immune Deficiency Foundation [8] on more than 1000 patients with PIDD, adverse reactions were observed in 44% of the patients. In the majority of cases these reactions were mild (back or abdominal aching or pain, nausea, rhinitis, asthma, chills, low grade fever, myalgias, headache). It is important to note, that in 34% of the patients the side effects emerged after the first administration of IVIG and after the following administrations the adverse effects became milder and fewer. The cessation of the IVIG infusion usually lead to fast resolution of the symptoms. The authors of the study recommend the administration of diphenhydramine, acetaminophen, aspirin, ibuprofen in such reactions, and in more severe cases – methylprednisolone 1 mg/kg b.w. and/or IV hydration with normal saline infusion. Some patient require pre-medication before the IVIG infusion.

Potentially Life-Threatening Side Effects of IVIG

IVIG could have some potentially life-threatening side effects, such as anaphylactic reactions, aseptic meningitis, acute renal failure, thromboembolic complications (stroke and myocardial infarction, pulmonary embolism), hemolysis, hepatitis, arthritis, et. [8]. The pathogenesis of these reactions remains unclear, yet hypersensitivity (immediate – IgE-mediated, and/or delayed), complement activation, cytokine release, direct irritation by the IVIG preparation and/or its adjuvants have been supposed to play roles in the development of these complications.

Anaphylactic Reactions

Severe anaphylactic reactions to IVIG have been observed mainly in patients with selective IgA immunoglobulin deficit with positive serum anti-IgA antibodies [14, 15]. The presence of traces of IgA in the IVIG infusion could lead to the formation of immune complexes containing IgA plus IgG and/or IgE anti-IgA antibodies [15], subsequent complement activation of reaction of immediate hypersensitivity (type I) and development of anaphylactic shock. These reactions are extremely rare, yet represent a life-threatening complication of IVIG treatment. For the period 1995-2007 S. Dashti-Khavidaki et al. [16] studied 99 patients with different forms of immune deficit who received a total of 3004 IVIG infusions and observed anaphylactic reactions in three (severe chest pain, severe wheezing and severe headache).

Thromboembolic Events

These complications have been described in elderly patients, with past history of coronary and cerebrovascular disease, in obese patients with diabetes mellitus, arterial hypertension, dyslipidemia, and in patients with hypovolemia and immobilization [7, 17-19], high doses of IVIG in rapid infusion rate. Following thromboembolic complications have been reported: myocardial infarction [20, 21], pulmonary embolism [22], stroke [23], deep venous thrombosis [24], etc. These complications are extremely rare [6] and are associated with different underlying conditions, such as platelet activation, increased plasma viscosity [7, 23], contamination of the IVIG with factor XIa [18].

Aseptic Meningitis

This complications of IVIG treatment has been observed in patients with history of migraine. The first signs and symptoms of aseptic meningitis develop within 24 hours of the IVIG infusion and last for 3-5 days – severe headache, meningism, photophobia, fever [14, 25, 26]. The examination of the cerebrospinal fluid reveals pleocytosis, eosinophylia, elevation of IgG levels [25]. This complication is very rare and develops mainly in high-dosed IVIG treatment with rapid infusion rate [26]. The pathogenesis of this complication remains unclear, but possible mechanisms include: hypersensitivity reaction, stabilizing products, release of cytokines, cerebrovascular sensitivity, and direct meningeal irritation by the drug and/or its adjuvants [27]. Though this reaction is thought to be a serious complication following IVIG therapy, it is usually self-limiting and manageable. On the other hand, it could be a source of dilemma for the clinician – whether the (aseptic) meningitis is associated with the treatment, or with the underlying disease – i.e., intracranial bleeding in ITP, infection in immunoglobulin deficits, HIV or leukemia [27]. As in thromboembolic complications and in acute renal failure post IVIG administration, the development of aseptic meningitis could be prevented with slow infusion rate and good hydration of the patient, especially in patients with well known risk for these complications [26, 27]. If aseptic meningitis develops, the best strategy is thought to be watchful waiting with sufficient hydration and steroid treatment is rarely required. In some cases, premedication with non-steroid anti-inflammatory drugs and/or antihistamines is advisable [27]. Other possible neurological complications of IVIG treatment described in the literature are: encephalopathy with seizures, migrainous headache, hypothermia [14].

Acute Renal Failure

This is a serious complication following IVIG treatment, especially in systemic autoimmune diseases with renal involvement. Renal impairment in

IVIG treatment is associated with the use of certain stabilizers, e.g., sucrose (due to the lack of sucrase in the kidney, accumulation in the proximal tubule and subsequent hyperosmolarity leading to renal injury – this condition is close to the so called "sucrose nephropathy", described in the past in patients infused with hypertonic sucrose solutions) [2, 14, 28]. Sucrose is uptaken by the renal proximal tubular epithelium by pinocytosis, incorporated in the lysosomes and causes intracellular hyperosmolarity, vacuolization of the cytoplasm, both cellular injury and "intratubular hydronephrosis" (due to cellular edema of the tubular epithelium and narrowing of tubular lumina) with decreased diuresis. Pseudohyponatriemia has also been described in these patients. This renal complication develops most frequently in patients with pre-existing/underlying renal disease, diabetes, in elderly, dehydration/volume depletion, sepsis, paraproteinemia, concomitant use of other nephrotoxic agents. The incidence of acute renal failure in IVIG preparations stabilized with other agents (i.e., glucose, mannitol, maltose, D-sorbitol, l-proline, glycine) is much lower [2, 28]. Other cause of acute renal failure during IVIG treatment include: acute tubulo-interstitial nephritis of allergic origin (IgE-mediated), complement activation in delayed hypersensitivity, acute renal injury in anaphylactic shock, etc.

Hemolysis

This is a severe and extremely reaction to IVIG treatment, associated with the presence of anti-A, anti-B and/or anti-D antibodies in the IVIG preparations (i.e., passive transfer of anti-A, anti-B or anti-D antibodies in IVIG), developing more frequently in pre-sensitized patients (e.g., poly-transfusion patients, renal and bone marrow transplant recipients, etc.) [29, 30]. Predisposing factors could be the presence of underlying inflammatory condition, low osmotic resistance of the red blood cells, underlying hemolytic anemia, etc. Neutropenia of immune origin has also been described.

Hepatitis and Arthritis

These two types of reactions to IVIG treatment are extremely rare, probably due to delayed hypersensitivity reactions, complement activation and/or cytokine release. Also, passive transfer of anti-HCV, anti-HBV and other antibodies has been described in patients treated with IVIG. As in IVIG-induced hemolysis, these complications could be mediated by passively transferred autoantibodies contained in the IVIG preparation. The clinician should be aware of this possibility of passive transfer of antiviral antibodies when investigating such patients.

Other more or less severe side effects of IVIG preparations include [14]:

- Hypotension (due to immunoglobulin dimmers in the preparation, activation of monocytes/macrophages, neutrophils, platelet activating factor [PAF]).
- Volume overload and/or pulmonary edema (the latter – due to volume overload or to increased pulmonary caplillary permeability or to the presence of high-titer ANCA).
- Dermatological complications – eczema.

Investigations That Should Be Performed Prior to the Administration of IVIG

Prior to the administration of IVIG following parameters should be investigated:

- Serum cryoglobulins (high IgG and low IgA);
- Rheumatoid factor (RF) and cryoglobulins, especially in pre-existing rash and/or arthralgia;
- Creatinine, urea/BUN;
- Dys/paraproteinemia;
- Hyperpolinemia;
- Blood glucose;
- Platelet count;
- Genetic markers of hypercoagulation (factor V Leiden mutation, MTHFR gene polymorphism, PAI, etc.) – *especially in pregnancy*;
- Autoantibodies – antinuclear (ANA), antiphospholipid, antiovarian, antithyroid – *especially in pregnancy*;
- NK-cells – *especially in pregnancy*;
- CD4/CD8 – decreased CD8 count with subsequently increased CD4/CD8 count – *especially in pregnancy*;

Following factors should be considered prior to the initiation of IVIG treatment:

- Patient's age – in elderly patients the risk of complications and adverse reactions is significantly increased. In female patients with reproductive problems, IVIG are more appropriate treatment in elder women, while in younger patients the genetic abnormalities have leading role.
- Is the patient indicated for this treatment and are there alternative approaches?
- The risk/benefit profile of the treatment in the individual patient.
- The atherosclerotic risk.
- The cardiovascular risk.
- The presence of hypercoagulation (inborn or acquired thrombophilic state).
- The presence of hyperviscosity and/or paraproteinemia.
- Prolonged immobilization.
- Hydration (the presence of volume depletion / dehydration or volume overload, congestive heart failure).
- The presence and compensation of diabetes.
- The presence of hypertriglyceridemia.
- The presence of sepsis with or without systemic response.
- Concomitant treatment with nephrotoxic agents and/or underlying renal disease.
- Which IVIG preparation should be chosen (whether the sucrose-containing preparations are suitable in the individual patient)?
- Careful evaluation in case preparation should be changed or the treatment dose should be altered.

Prior to the initiation of IVIG treatment the clinician should be familiar with the characteristics of the individual IVIG preparation – each preparation contains pooled immunoglobulins from multiple donors, including different antibodies that undergo different methods for viral inactivation, purification, stabilization; the individual preparations differ in pH, IgA content, stabilizing agent, salt content, osmolality and could potentially cause different side effects.

During the IVIG infusion following factors should be considered: close monitoring of patient's vital signs (every 15 minutes during the first hour of the infusion and hourly afterwards), the infusion should be performed in hospitals or in day care centers. The patient should not receive life vaccines 2 weeks before and 3 month after the administration of IVIG. Prior to the administration of IVIG informed consent should be received from the patient and/or his/her legal representative. The risk of infectious complications should also be considered. And, last but not least, comes the question *Who will pay for this expensive treatment?*

Causes for the development of adverse reactions to IVIG

- Improper use (wrong diagnosis and/or wrong patient).
- Insufficient pre- and post-treatment investigations (biochemical, hematological, immunological).
- High rate and/or high quantity of IVIG infused in a short time (1.2-2.0 g/kg b.w. for 1-2 hours, for 3-5 successive days), frequent administration (≤14 days).
- Lack of/insufficient monitoring during and after the infusion.
- IVIG adjuvants, stabilizers, etc.
- Sucrose.
- Aggregates in the IVIG preparation (dimeric and polymeric immunoglobulins) that could lead to degranulation of neutrophils.
- Traces of IgA (especially in patients with *selective IgA deficiency).*
- Presence of ANCA in titers from 1:32 to 1:2048 (directed against lactoferrin, leukocyte elastase, catepsin, bactericidal/permeability increasing protein, but not against myeloperoxidase and serin protease) in the IVIG preparation.
- The presence of ANA in titers 1:30-1:240 in the IVIG preparation.
- The presence of anti-smooth-muscle antibodies (ASMA) in certain IVIG preparations in titer 1:240. These autoantibodies do not have anti-actin activity (that could lead to interference with ANCA contained in the IVIG preparations).
- The stated autoantibodies (ANCA, ANA, ASMA) are found in low titers in the sera of healthy people (natural autoantibodies) but in pooled IVIG preparations their titers could increase significantly and they could target natural self-antigens. In massive IVIG infusion these "natural autoantibodies" cannot be blocked by the recipient.
- The natural reaction of the human body to infusion of large doses of IVIG is due to the response to immunoglobulin aggregates, to large

quantities of antibodies initiating immune response, oxidative burst, PAF activation, degranulation of certain cells (especially neutrophils).

- Last but not least, the clinician should not forget the risk of transmissive infection (HIV, hepatitis B and C, etc.). Nowadays, after the development of screening tests and of virus-inactivating agents, the risk of such complications is much lower than in the past. Still, the risk of Creutzfeld-Jakobs disease should not be underestimated, especially in regions with high prevalence of the disease. Passive transfer of anti-viral antibodies with the infusion of IVIG has been described, including antibodies against HIV, hepatitis B and C virus. The clinician should be aware of the latter phenomenon when evaluating patients on IVIG treatment.

Treatment of the IVIG-Associated Adverse Reactions

As stated above, the treatment and prevention of IVIG-related side-effects consists in: proper evaluation of the patient and the IVIG preparation, premedication with non-steroid anti-inflammatory drugs and/or antihistamines, treatment of allergic and/or immune mediated reactions with corticosteroids, antihistamines, epinephrine, and supportive treatment (including proper water and electrolyte balance, dialysis if required).

Conclusion

IVIG treatment has saved thousands of lives and has improved the quality of life of many patients with immune deficiencies, autoimmune and infectious diseases. The wider use of these preparations has lead to the emergence of some rare and potentially lethal side effects, such as aseptic meningitis, hemolytic anemia, acute renal failure and thrombo-embolic incidents. Therefore, careful evaluation of the patient, the therapeutic indications and the IVIG preparations and concomitant treatment is needed prior to the initiation of IVIG therapy.

References

[1] Ibanez, C; Montoro-Ronsano, JM. Intravenous immunoglobulin preparations and autoimmune disorders: mechanisms of action. *Curr Pharm Biotechnol*, 2003, 4, 239-47.

[2] Dantal, J. Intravenous Immunoglobulins: In-Depth Review of Excipiens and acute kidney injury risk. *Am J Nephrol*, 2013, 38, 275-284.

[3] Orange, JS; Hassny, EM; Weiler, CR;Ballow; et al. Use of intravenous immunoglobulin in human disease: A review of evidence by members of the Primary Immunodeficiency Committee of the American Academy of Allergy, Asthma and Immunology. *J Allergy ClinImmunol*, 2006, 117, S525-53.

[4] Gelfand, EW. Intravenous immune globulin in autoimmune and inflammatory diseases. *N Engl J Med*, 2012, 367, 2015-2025.

[5] Leong, H; Stachnik, J; Bonk, ME; Matuszewski, KA. Unlabeled uses of intravenous immune globulin. *Am J Health Syst Pharm*, 2008, 65, 1815-1824.

[6] Brennan, VM; Salome-Bentley, NJ; Chapel, HM. Prospectiveaudit of adverse reactions occurring in 459 primaryantibody-deficient patients receiving intravenous immunoglobulin. *Clin Exp Immunol*, 2003, 133, 247–251.

[7] Katz, U; Achiron, A; Sherer, Y; Shoenfeld, Y. Safety of intravenousimmunoglobulin (IVIG) therapy. *Autoimmun Rev*, 2007, 6, 257–259.

[8] 2002 Immune Deficiency Foundation patient survey. http://www.primaryimmune.org/pidsurvey.htm. Accessed November 2005.

[9] Wimperis, J; Lunn, M; Jones, A; et al.: *Clinicalguidelines for immunoglobulin use*, Secondedition update, 2011. http://www.dh.gov.uk/prod_consum_dh/groups/dh_digitalassets/documents/digitalasset/dh_131107.pdf (accessedSeptember 21, 2012).

[10] Agence Nationale de Sécurité du Médicamentet des Produits de Santé: Octagam 100 mg/ml, solution pour perfusion. http://ansm.sante.fr/Dossiers-thematiques/Referentiels-de-bonusage-des-medicaments/Immunoglobulines/Tableau-immunoglobulines/OCTAGAM-100-mg-ml-solution-pour-perfusion (accessed September 21, 2012).

[11] Anderson, D; Ali, K; Blanchette, V; et al.: Guidelineson the use of intravenous immune globulinfor hematologic conditions. *TransfusMed Rev*, 2007, 21(suppl 1),S9–S56.

[12] Feasby, T; Banwell, B; Benstead, T; et al.: Guidelineson the use of intravenous immune globulinfor neurologic conditions. *Transfus MedRev*, 2007, 21(suppl 1),S57–S107.
[13] Group APIIE. Consensus recommendationsfor the use of immunoglobulin replacementtherapy in immune deficiency. 2009. http://www.info4pi.org/Documents/Publications/APIIEG%20Consensus%20Recommendations%20Edition%202%20July%202009_20120201_170745.pdf (accessed September21, 2012).
[14] Knezevic-Maramica, I; Kruskall, MS. Intravenous immune globulins: an update for clinicians. *Transfusion*, 2003, 43, 1460-1480.
[15] deAlbuquerque Campos, R; Sato, MN; daSilva Duarte, AJ. IgGantiIgA subclasses in common variable immunodeficiency and association with severe adverse reactions to intravenous immunoglobulin therapy *JClinImmunol*, 2000, 20 (1), 77-82.
[16] Dashti-Khavidaki, S; Aghamohammadi,A; Farshadi,F; Mavahedi,M; et al. Adverse reactions of prophylactic intravenousimmunoglobulin; A 13-year experience with 3004 infusions in Iranian patients with primary immunodeficiency diseases. *J Invest AllergolClinImmunol*, 2009, 19 (2), 139-145.
[17] Liumbruno, G; Bennardello, F; Lattanzio, A; Piccolo, P; Rossetti, G. Recommendation for the use of albumin and immunoglobulins. *Blood Transfus*, 2009, 7, 216-234.
[18] Wolfberg, AS; Kon, RH; Monroe, DM; Hoffman, M. Coagulation factor XI is a contaminant in intravenous immunoglobulin preparations. *Am J Hematol*, 2000, 65 (1), 30-34.
[19] Hefer, D; Jaloudi, M. Thromboembolic events as an emerging adverse effect during high-dose intravenous immunoglobulin therapy in elderly patients: a case report and discussion of the relevant literature. *Ann Hematol*, 2005, 84, 411-415.
[20] Elkayam, O;Paran, D; Milo, R; et al. Acute myocardial infarction associated with high dose intravenous immunoglobulin infusion for autoimmune disorders: a study of four cases. *Ann Rheum Dis*, 2000, 59, 77-80.
[21] Paolini, R; Fabris, F;Cella, G. Acute myocardial infarction during treatment with intravenous immunoglobulin for idiopathic thrombocytopenic purpura (ITP). *Am J Hematol*, 2000, 65, 177-6.
[22] Alliot, C; Rapin, JP;Besson, M; et al. Pulmonary embolism after intravenous immunoglobulin. *J Royal Soc Med*, 2001, 94, 187-8.

[23] Dalakas, MC. Intravenous immunoglobulin in autoimmune neuromuscular diseases. *JAMA*, 2004, 291 (10), 2367-2375.

[24] Go, RS; Calli, TG. Deepvenousthrombosis of the arm after intravenous immunoglobulin infusion: case report and literature review of intravenous immunoglobulin-related thrombotic complications. *Mayo ClinProc*, 2000, 75, 83-5.

[25] Sekul, EA; Cupler, EJ; Dalakas, MC. Aseptic Meningitis Associated with High-Dose Intravenous Immunoglobulin Therapy: Frequency and Risk Factors. *Ann Intern Med,* 1994,121(4),259-262.

[26] Katz, U; Achiron, A; Sherer, Y; Shoenfeld, Y. Safety of intravenous immunoglobulin (IVIG) therapy. *Autoimm Rev*, 2007, 6(4), 257-9.

[27] Kaarthigeyan, K;B urli, VV. Aseptic meningitis following intravenous immunoglobulin therapy of common variable immunodeficiency. *J PediatrNeurosci*, 2011,6(2),160–161.

[28] Ippoliti, C; Williams, LA; Huber, S. Toxicity of rapidly infused andconcentrated immune globulin. *ClinPharmacol*, 1992, 11, 1022-1026.

[29] Kahwaji, J; Barker, E; Pepkowitz, S; et al. Acute hemolysis after high-dose intravenous immunoglobulin therapy in highly HLA sensitized patients. *Clin J Am SocNephrol*, 2009,4,1993-1997.

[30] Pintova, S; Bhardwaj, A;Aledort, LM. IVIG – a hemolytic culprit.*N Engl J Med*, 2012, 367,974-976.

In: Plasmapheresis and Intravenous … ISBN: 978-1-63117-916-7
Editor: Rossana Allegro

Chapter 9

THERAPEUTIC PLASMA EXCHANGE IN THE NEUROLOGICAL SETTING: SOME SPECIAL CASES

Karin Janssen van Doorn, MD[1,*] and Sanne Vellinga, MD[2]

[1]Department of Nephrology-Hypertension, Antwerp University Hospital, Belgium
[2]Department of Intensive Care, Erasmus University Rotterdam, The Netherlands

INTRODUCTION

Therapeutic Plasma Exchange (TPE) is a therapeutic procedure in which blood of the patient is passed through a medical device, which separates plasma from the blood components. TPE is designed to remove or at least to reduce the concentration of (pathologic) large molecular weight substances from the plasma. The idea behind the procedure is that elimination of pathologic substances from the plasma reduces further physiological damage. TPE is mostly not a solitude therapeutic intervention to stop a pathological process, and is often accompanied with orally or intravenous drugs.

* E-mail: karin.janssen.van.doorn@uza.be; Phone: +32/3/821-3421; Fax: +32/3/829-0100.

Therefore, it is interesting to know the pathologic substance, because it should be toxic, larger than 15000 Dalton, with a long half-life, to make removal by plasmapheresis in stead of other eliminating techniques as hemofiltration or high-flux hemodialysis, valuable.

The best known indications in the neurological setting are Myastenia Gravis and Guillain Barré syndrome [1]. When TPE is used in neurological disorders, there is not always certainty about the pathogenic substance that triggers the development of the disease. Mostly an autoimmune pathogenesis is suggested due to the presence of antibodies. The presumed antibody mediated tissue damage could probably interrupted by TPE.

Nowadays, evidence-based medicine is practiced and the ASFA guidelines promote therapeutic apheresis based on clinical data and controlled trials, rather than case reports. Indications are divided in different categories, based on evidence of clinical efficacy [1, 2], ongoing from category I, disorders for which apheresis is accepted as first-line therapy, (for instance Guillain-Barré syndrome); category II for second-line therapy, (e.g acute disseminated encephalomyelitis); category III, in which the role of apheresis is not confirmed (paraneoplastic neurologic syndrome) to category IV, including disorders for which apheresis should be ineffective or harmful [1]. There is a seperate category in which apheresis is only used in an experimental setting.

Although, the quality of evidence supporting the use of TPE in the treatment of most neurological diseases and disorders is often limited and many of the conditions are rare, it is unlikely that randomized controlled trials (RCT) will ever be performed [1]. Therefore, we retrospectively examined all adult TPE-patients during a 7-year period (March 2005 - February 2012) and discovered some interesting observations [3].

Study Design

Retrospectively available data on patient characteristics, their indication for TPE, the level of evidence for every indication, additional treatment, result of treatment and survival were obtained from our central patient data system. Partial response to treatment was defined as amelioration of clinical and/or laboratory measures. Complete response was defined as complete recovery of clinical and relevant laboratory measures. We also documented the number of TPE sessions and the number of episodes of TPE (defined as a new series of sessions at least one month after the last session). Indications and level of evidence were determined according to the definitions and guidelines on the use of therapeutic apheresis published by the American Society for Apheresis (ASFA) in 2010 [1].

During this period 69 patients were included, of whom 52.2% were male and mean age at the first session was 51.8 (± 18,0) years. Mean number of treatment episodes was 1.3 (range 1-7, median 1) and mean number of TPE sessions was 9.0 (range 1-140, median 5). In 41 patients (59.4%) TPE was performed based on a level I indication, in 14 (20.3%) there was a level II indication, in 8 (11.6%) a level III indication, whereas one patient had a level IV indication (1.4%) and 5 patients suffered from a condition that was not included in the guidelines (7.2%). Forty patients were treated by TPE, because of a neurological disorder. These neurological diseases and their frequencies are reported in table 1 together with the level of evidence considering the indication for TPE. Patients off-category are indicated by an asterix.

We found no trend in number of treatments per year, or distribution, or category of indication (data not shown). A complete response was observed in 17 patients of the total population (24.6%). A partial response was seen in 42 patients (60.9%) and 10 patients (14.5%) experienced no response. During a follow-up period of 4 to 89 months, 18 patients (26.1%) died. When considering categories of indication we found no difference in response (100% no indication versus 85.7% category I-III, $p = 0.35$), probably because of the small number of patients with condition not rated in the guidelines. When these five (four neurological, one nephrological) patients, with a diagnosis not mentioned in the guidelines are excluded, the response rate is inversely correlated with the level of evidence (category I 97.6%, category II 71.4%, category III 50%, category IV 0% response, $p < 0.01$) [3].

DISCUSSION

In our population we see no trend in change of frequency or class of indication over the years. Most indications for TPE are of nephrologic or neurologic diagnostic origin. The distribution of indications is similar as reported in the studies of Lankford et al. [4] and Yeo et al. [5].

Considering non-rated conditions autoimmune limbic encephalitis is thought to be a channelopathy and a potential reversible component was suggested. Although several treatment algorithms implement TPE, there is no randomized controlled trial evidence [6, 7]. Evaluation of clinical evolution is partially based on subjective measures, which complicate the evaluation of treatment.

Table 1. Diagnosis and level of evidence

		Level of evidence	
Diagnosis	Frequency	Category	Grade
Acute disseminated encephalomyelitis (ADEM)	2	II	2c
Acute inflammatory demyelinating polyneuropathy (Guillain Barré syndrome)	1	I	1a
Autoimmune limbic encephalitis*	1	-	-
Myasthenia gravis moderate-severe	27	I	1a
Multifocal motor neuropathy*	1	-	-
Transverse myelitis	1	II	1c
Neuromyeltis optica	1	II	1c
Opsoclonus and gait ataxia*	1	-	-
Paraneoplastic neurologic syndrome	3	III	2c
Neuromyotonia (Isaacs' syndrome)*	1	-	-
Phytanic acid storage disease (Refsum's disease)	1	III	2c

As for multifocal motor neuropathy the underlying pathological mechanisms are unclear, but IgM autoantibodies against the ganglioside GM1 may cause changes in nodal and perinodal structures that compromise nerve conduction. Prednisolone and plasmapheresis are ineffective in most patients and may even exacerbate symptoms and are therefore not recommended [8]. Still in our patient we did see an, albeit again subjective, amelioration of complaints.

Neuromyotonia is another autoimmune channelopathy and TPE has been described as a second line therapy after anticonvulsants [7]. As for the case of the patient with opsoclonus and gait ataxia no clear evidence was found. All cases considering non-rated indications had a favorable outcome, which suggests that although without good evidence, in individual cases and after careful evaluation of indication and possible risks TPE can be of benefit. Main problem with these diseases is the fact that many complaints can only be measured subjectively and treatment never consisted of TPE alone.

Transverse Myelitis describes a heterogeneous group of inflammatory disorders that may arise from various causes, but it most often occurs in an autoimmune phenomenon after an infection or vaccination or as a result of an underlying systemic autoimmune disease, or an acquired demyelinating disease such as multiple sclerosis or the spectrum of disorders related to neuromyelitis optica [9]. In our series Transverse Myelitis was classified as neuromyelitis optica, but factual it is not classified in the ASFA guidelines. However, the patient with Transverse Myelitis also showed an optimal response and her outcome was classified as 'good' after TPE.

Our data were reviewed using the ASFA guidelines and although recent and well documented when concerning scientific evidence, a possible flaw is that the committee behind these guidelines includes physicians with training in pathology, hematology and pediatrics but not in nephrology or neurology. As such nephrologists are regularly confronted with a dilemma when not making the primary diagnosis but still being responsible for performing the definitive therapy, with all its attendant risks [5].

CONCLUSION

Besides well-known indications for TPE with strong evidence, for many diseases the indication for TPE is controversial or even obscure. In our population the response rate is indeed inversely correlated with the level of evidence, but only after exclusion of the patients with a diagnosis not mentioned in the guidelines. We suggest that controversial neurological indications are carefully evaluated on an individual base and a trial of TPE cannot be solely ruled out because of lack of evidence. Besides, it is worthwhile to publish case reports with positive or negative clinical evolution after TPE used in individually cases. It is important that in these settings careful and multidisciplinary review of all determining factors is obligatory.

REFERENCES

[1] Szczepiorkowski Z. M., Winters J. L., Bandarenko N., Kim H. C., Linenberger M. L., Marques M. B., Sarode R., Schwartz J., Weinstein R., Shaz B. H. Guidelines on the use of therapeutic apheresis in clinical practice: evidence-based approach from the Apheresis Applications

Committee of the American Society for Apheresis. *J. Clin. Apher.*, 2010;25:83-177.

[2] Winters J. L. Apheresis medicine. *J. Clin. Apher.*, 2011;26:239-242.

[3] Vellinga S., Verpooten G. A., Janssen van Doorn K. Trends in therapeutic plasma exchange: a single center evaluation. *Int. J. Artif. Organs,* 2013;36:730-737.

[4] Lankford K. V., Grindon A. J., Lyles R. H., Hillyer C. D. Indications for therapeutic plasma exchange at a university hospital and a regional blood center. *J. Clin. Apher.,* 2000;15:242-248.

[5] Yeo F. E., Bohen E. M., Yuan C. M., Sawyers E. S., Abbott K. C. Therapeutic plasma exchange as a nephrological procedure: a Single-Center Experience. *J. Clin. Apher.,* 2005;20:208-216.

[6] Bazir Ahmad S. A., Archer H. A., Ricel C. M., Gerhand S., Bradly M., Wilkins A. Seronegative limbic encephalitis: case report, literature review and proposed treatment algorithm. *Pract. Neurol.*, 2011;11:355-361.

[7] Michaud M., Delrieu J., Astudillo L. Autoimmune channelopathies. *Rev. Med. Int.,* 2011;32:742-750.

[8] Vlam L., van der Pol W. L., Cats E. A., Straver D. C., Piepers S., Franssen H., van den Berg L. H. Multifocal motor neuropathy: diagnosis, pathogenesis and treatment strategies. *Nat. Rev. Neurol.,* 2012;8:48.

[9] Frohman E. M., Wingerchuk D. M. Transverse Myelitis. N. Engl. J. Med., 2010;363:564-72.

INDEX

B

C

F

G

H

I

J

N

O

P

Q

R

S

T

U

V

W

Y